diabetes

JODY VASSALLO

FORTIORI

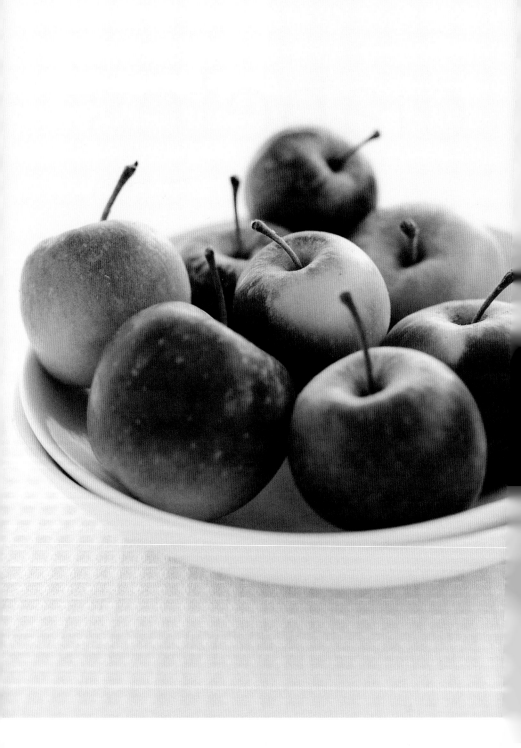

ABOUT DIABETES

On average, almost ten per cent of the population in western countries have diabetes and unfortunately this number continues to rise. But there are steps anyone can take to either reduce the risk of developing the disease; control the disease once it is diagnosed; or possibly even reverse the condition. In the past, diets for diabetics were relatively limited and often stressful. Thanks to scientific research, it is now known that a diabetic diet does not have to be so stringent, and moderate amounts of sweet foods can usually be included. A low-fat diet based on low-GI, carbohydrate-rich foods is an important part of the recommended therapy for people with diabetes. This book provides diabetics with general guidelines for healthy eating and contains delicious recipes to assist in achieving these goals. The recipes are also nutritionally analysed and GI-rated. However, the information in this book should not replace any advice given to you by a doctor or dietitian. Your individual health needs may require specific dietary restrictions or changes, so check with both your doctor and dietitian before making any changes to your diet, exercise habits or medication to make sure that they are safe for you.

Dr Susanna Holt
(PhD and registered dietitian)

WHAT IS DIABETES?

Diabetes is a condition in which the blood sugar (glucose) level is excessively high for one of two reasons: either the body cannot produce enough insulin, or the body cannot use insulin properly. In both healthy people and diabetics, blood sugar rises after eating as the food's carbohydrates are digested into glucose and absorbed into the blood. In healthy people, the rise in blood sugar stimulates the pancreas to release a hormone called insulin. Insulin enables body cells to absorb the glucose and fats in the blood, causing the blood sugar level to fall back down to normal. In people with diabetes, the pancreas doesn't make enough insulin or the cells don't respond to it properly, so glucose and fats cannot get into the body's cells and build up in the blood. The blood sugar rises to a higher level after eating, doesn't fall as quickly, and remains higher than normal, even many hours after eating. If left untreated, the high blood glucose and fat levels can damage the eyes, nerves and blood vessels, and increase the risk of heart disease, kidney and circulatory problems. Symptoms of undiagnosed diabetes can include frequent urination, excessive thirst, tiredness, infections and leg cramps. Early diagnosis and appropriate treatment are an essential part of minimising the risk of the serious health problems associated with diabetes.

TYPES OF DIABETES

There are three main types of diabetes and a pre-diabetic condition:

1 | **Type 1 (insulin-dependent or juvenile-onset diabetes)** - is the most serious but least common form and mostly occurs in normal weight children and young adults. People with type 1 diabetes cannot make the hormone insulin due to a damaged pancreas and require daily insulin injections to stay alive.

2 | **Type 2 (non-insulin dependent or adult-onset diabetes)** - is the most common form and usually develops in overweight people after the age of 40 due to the body not responding to insulin properly. The risk of developing type 2 diabetes is increased by being overweight and inactive, having a family history of diabetes, and eating too much fat and refined carbohydrates. Treatment revolves around healthy eating, weight control and physical activity.

3 | **Gestational** - is a temporary form of diabetes that develops in some women during pregnancy because certain hormones stop insulin from working properly. It usually disappears once the pregnancy is over, but if left untreated can result in a difficult delivery and health problems in the infant. It is usually detected during a routine blood test at 24-28 weeks, and is generally treated with healthy eating alone. Gestational diabetes increases the risk of developing type 2 diabetes later in life, but this can be reduced with a healthy lifestyle.

Impaired glucose tolerance (IGT) - is a pre-diabetic condition where blood glucose is higher than normal but not in the diabetic range. IGT increases the risk of developing type 2 diabetes but this can be prevented with a healthy diet and regular exercise, both of which are more effective than medication. As little as 30 minutes a day of moderate physical activity, such as brisk walking, coupled with some weight loss, will improve your health.

MANAGING DIABETES

The main goal is to keep blood glucose within a relatively normal range to prevent problems such as heart disease, kidney failure, and blindness. Diabetes is a long-term problem, so you will need to make lifestyle changes and learn to monitor your condition by:

1 | eating a healthy diet and maintaining a healthy weight

2 | getting regular physical activity and reducing stress levels

3 | taking any diabetes-related medication prescribed for you

4 | not smoking and only drinking alcohol in moderation, if at all

5 | regularly checking your blood sugar

6 | consulting your doctor and other relevant health professionals.

STEPS TO HEALTHY EATING

1 | Eat low-GI, carbohydrate-rich meals

Eating 4-6 smaller carbohydrate-rich meals and snacks, spread over the day, rather than 2-3 large meals will help control blood glucose. Ask your dietitian for advice about scheduling food intake around medication and activity patterns. Monitoring your blood glucose will also help you find out when and what you should eat, or if you've eaten too much.

2 | Limit total fat (particularly saturated fat)

Eating too much saturated fat can cause weight gain, poor blood glucose control and high blood cholesterol, all of which are known to increase the risk of heart disease. Try to use low-fat cooking methods and choose low-fat dairy products, lean meat and poultry, and low-fat spreads. Limit your intake of fried and fast foods, biscuits, pastries and cakes. Use small amounts of canola or olive oil when cooking and eat oily fish 2-3 times each week to make sure you get enough healthy essential omega-3 fats.

3 | Increase fruit and vegetable intake

Aim to eat at least 2 serves of fruit and 5 serves of vegetables each day. They will help you feel full, and in addition they contain many healthy nutrients, including antioxidants that can help protect tissues from being damaged by excess blood glucose.

4 | Limit sugar and sugary food intake

Sugar doesn't cause diabetes and people with well-controlled diabetes don't have to avoid sugar completely but it should be treated with caution, especially if you need to lose weight. Adding a little sugar (or, better still, fresh fruit) to a bowl of porridge or bran cereal won't raise blood sugar very much, but having a soft drink or lollies in between meals will send it soaring. Reduced-sugar products are readily available and provide sweetness without too many calories or raising blood sugar.

5 | Limit salt intake

Excess salt raises blood pressure, which increases the risk of heart and kidney disease. Avoid adding salt to meals and look for reduced- or no-added salt versions of canned and packaged foods. Use herbs, spices, lemon juice and vinegar for flavour.

6 | Limit alcohol intake

Alcohol is high in calories so avoid it if you are trying to lose weight or have poorly controlled diabetes. Health authorities recommend drinking a maximum of 1-2 standard drinks a day, with alcohol-free days each week. Choosing low-alcohol beer or diluting wine and spirits with soda water or a diet soft drink are better choices. If you take diabetic medication, you must eat some carbohydrate (such as bread or low-fat crackers) whenever you drink alcohol to reduce the risk of hypoglycaemia.

THE GI GUIDE

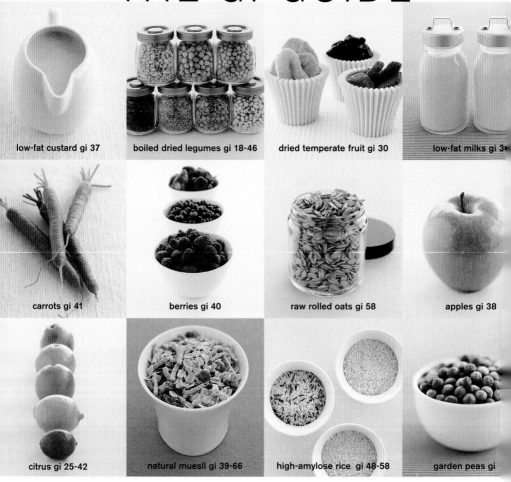

low-fat custard gi 37

boiled dried legumes gi 18-46

dried temperate fruit gi 30

low-fat milks gi 3

carrots gi 41

berries gi 40

raw rolled oats gi 58

apples gi 38

citrus gi 25-42

natural muesli gi 39-66

high-amylose rice gi 48-58

garden peas gi

Not all carbohydrates cause a blood sugar spike. In fact, the amount of sugar or starch in a food is not a good indication of its blood glucose (glycaemic) effect. There are many different types of sugars and starches, and they are digested at different rates and have different effects on blood glucose. Preparation and cooking methods will also affect the blood glucose response. The more processed a food is, the easier it is to digest and the higher its glycaemic index (GI) value. Scientists developed the GI method to measure the extent to which different carbohydrate-rich foods increase blood glucose when eaten.

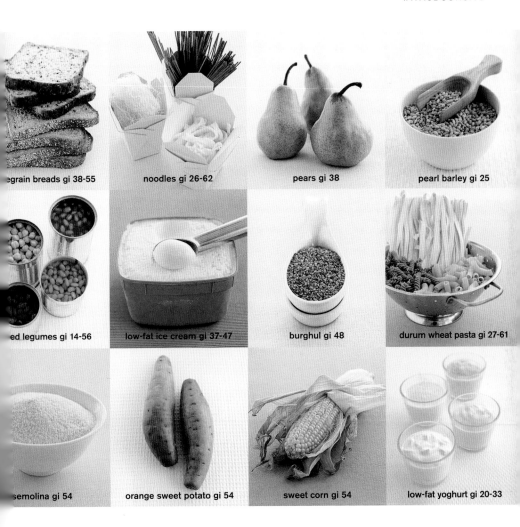

egrain breads gi 38-55 | noodles gi 26-62 | pears gi 38 | pearl barley gi 25

ed legumes gi 14-56 | low-fat ice cream gi 37-47 | burghul gi 48 | durum wheat pasta gi 27-61

semolina gi 54 | orange sweet potato gi 54 | sweet corn gi 54 | low-fat yoghurt gi 20-33

Although they contain the same amounts of carbohydrate, foods with a high GI value (>70) are digested faster and produce a quicker and higher rise in blood glucose than foods with a medium (56-69) or low GI value (<55). People with diabetes should choose carbohydrate-rich foods with low to medium GI values. Switching from high- to low-GI foods, limiting fat intake and exercising regularly will improve your health. At the end of every recipe in this book is a list of the nutrients contained in each serve of the dish, as well as its estimated GI value. For more GI information see www.glycemicindex.com

BREAKFAST

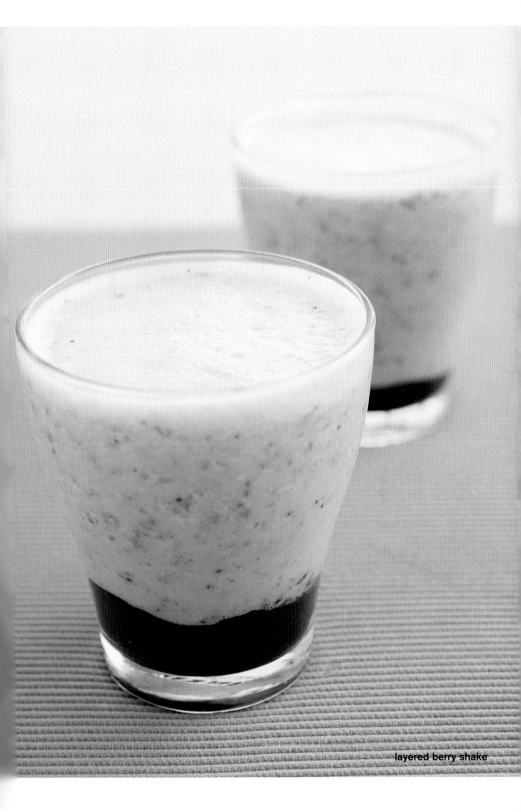

layered berry shake

LAYERED BERRY SHAKE

200 g (6½ oz) fresh
  or frozen raspberries
200 g (6½ oz) strawberries
1 (100 g/3⅓ oz) banana
2 tablespoons oat bran
1 (15 g/½ oz) wheat biscuit
1 tablespoon honey
2 tablespoons no-fat, no-added
  sugar vanilla yoghurt
2 cups (500 ml/16 fl oz) skim
  or no-fat milk

1 Put the raspberries into a blender and blend until smooth. Divide the puree among 4 glasses.
2 Put the remaining ingredients into the blender and blend until thick and creamy.
3 Carefully pour over the raspberry puree to form 2 separate layers. Serves 4

per serve ⏐ fat 1 g ⏐ protein 9.5 g ⏐ carbohydrate 28 g ⏐ fibre 5.5 g ⏐ cholesterol 6 mg ⏐ energy 725 kj (175 cal) ⏐ gi 41 ▼ low

OAT PORRIDGE WITH CARAMELISED APPLES

1 cup (95 g/3 oz) raw rolled oats
¼ cup (30 g/1 oz) semolina
2 tablespoons unprocessed
  oat bran
1 teaspoon vanilla essence
3 cups (750 ml/24 fl oz) water
10 g (⅓ oz) reduced-fat
  polyunsaturated margarine
2 medium red apples, unpeeled
  and cut into rounds
½ teaspoon ground cinnamon
½ cup (125 ml/4 fl oz)
  unsweetened apple juice
1 cup (250 ml/8 fl oz)
  reduced-fat milk

1 Put the rolled oats, semolina, oat bran, vanilla and water into a pan and cook over medium heat for 5-10 minutes, stirring occasionally until the porridge is thick and creamy.
2 Heat the margarine in a non-stick fry pan, add the apples and cinnamon and cook over medium heat until the apples are browned on both sides.
3 Add the apple juice and cook over high heat until the liquid has evaporated and the apples are soft.
4 Spoon the porridge into bowls, top with the milk and finish with the caramelised apples. Serves 4

per serve ⏐ fat 4 g ⏐ protein 7 g ⏐ carbohydrate 40 g ⏐ fibre 4.5 g ⏐ cholesterol 2 mg ⏐ energy 940 kj (225 cal) ⏐ gi 43 ▼ low

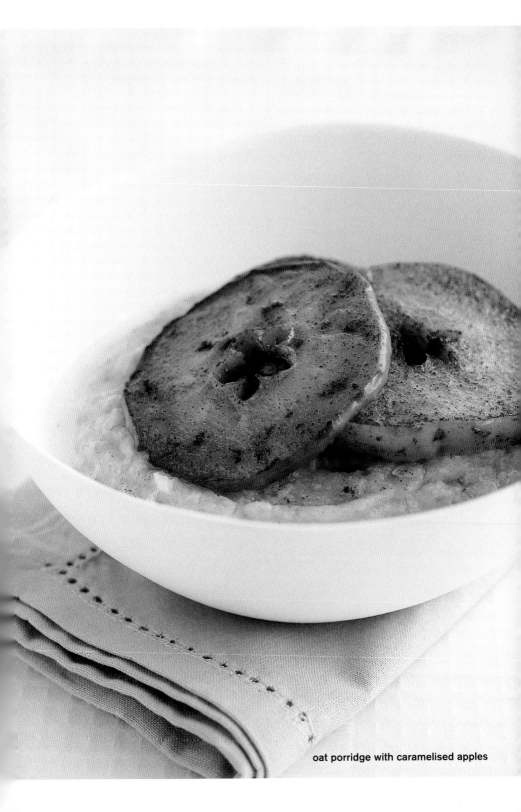

oat porridge with caramelised apples

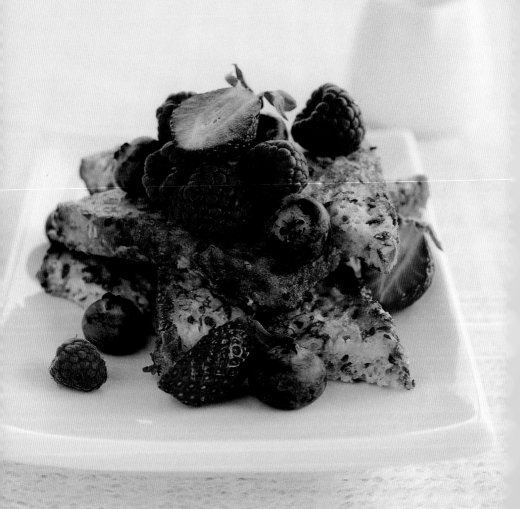

french toast with berries & yoghurt

FRENCH TOAST WITH BERRIES & YOGHURT

1 Whisk together the eggs, milk and sugar or sweetener and dip the bread, one slice at a time, into the egg mixture.

2 Heat a non-stick fry pan over medium heat and cook the bread until the egg has set and the bread is golden brown on both sides. Keep the finished slices warm while the remaining slices are cooked.

3 Serve stacks of the bread topped with yoghurt and berries. Serves 4

per serve (sugar) | fat 5 g | protein 19 g | carbohydrate 48.5 g | fibre 5 g | cholesterol 103.5 mg | energy 1320 kj (315 cal) | gi 40 ▼ low

per serve (sweetener) | fat 5 g | protein 19 g | carbohydrate 41 g | fibre 5 g | cholesterol 103.5 mg | energy 1205 kj (290 cal) | gi 33 ▼ low

2 eggs, lightly beaten

1 cup (250 ml/8 fl oz) skim or no-fat milk

2 tablespoons sugar or low-calorie sweetener suitable for cooking

8 slices (320 g/10²/₃ oz) grainy soy and linseed bread

400 ml (13 fl oz) no-fat, no-added sugar vanilla yoghurt

300 g (10 oz) mixed fresh or frozen berries

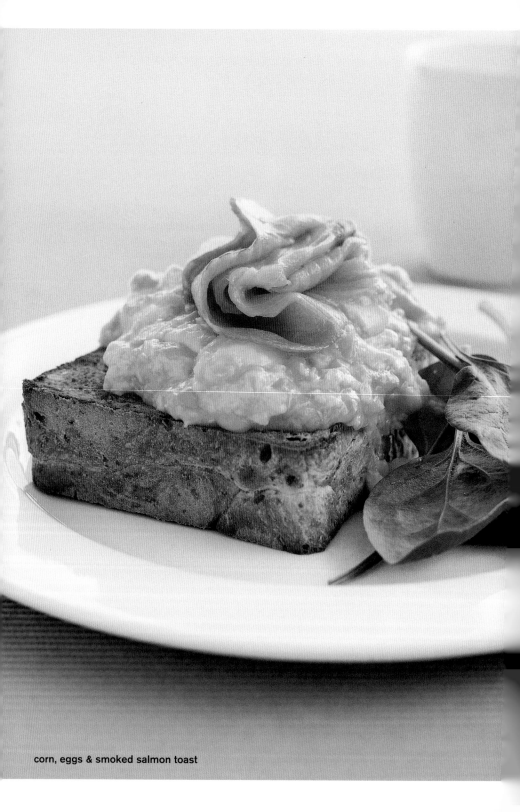

corn, eggs & smoked salmon toast

CORN, EGGS & SMOKED SALMON TOAST

1 Cut the bread into 4 x 2.5 cm (1 in) thick slices, toast and spread it with margarine.

2 Whisk the eggs and milk together and cook in a non-stick fry pan over medium heat. Stir until the eggs just begin to scramble, then stir in the creamed corn.

3 Cook for 3 minutes or until heated through. Season with cracked black pepper. Serve the toast topped with eggs, corn and smoked salmon. Serve the spinach to the side. Serves 4

per serve | fat 10.5 g | protein 24 g | carbohydrate 52.5 g | fibre 7.5 g | cholesterol 201 mg | energy 1680 kj (400 cal) | gi 48 ▼ low

1 small loaf (345 g/11½ oz) wholegrain bread
10 g (⅓ oz) reduced-fat polyunsaturated margarine
4 eggs, lightly beaten
¾ cup (185 ml/6 fl oz) skim or no-fat milk
310 g (10 oz) can creamed corn
cracked black pepper
100 g (3⅓ oz) smoked salmon
100 g (3⅓ oz) baby spinach

SPICED COUSCOUS, FRUIT COMPOTE & YOGHURT

1 Put the couscous, dried fruit salad, cranberries and pistachio nuts into a bowl.

2 Heat the milk, cinnamon and cardamom in a pan and bring just to the boil. Pour the milk over the couscous and allow to stand for 10 minutes or until the liquid has been absorbed.

3 Remove the cinnamon and cardamom and serve bowls of couscous, topped with yoghurt. Serves 6

per serve | fat 3 g | protein 11 g | carbohydrate 73 g | fibre 5.5 g | cholesterol 5.5 mg | energy 1515 kj (360 cal) | gi 45 ▼ low

1 cup (180 g/6 oz) couscous
300 g (10 oz) dried fruit salad, roughly chopped
100 g (3⅓ oz) dried cranberries
30 g (1 oz) pistachio nuts, roughly chopped
2 cups (500 ml/16 fl oz) skim or no-fat milk
1 cinnamon stick
4 cardamom pods, bruised
200 ml (6½ fl oz) no-fat, no-added sugar vanilla yoghurt

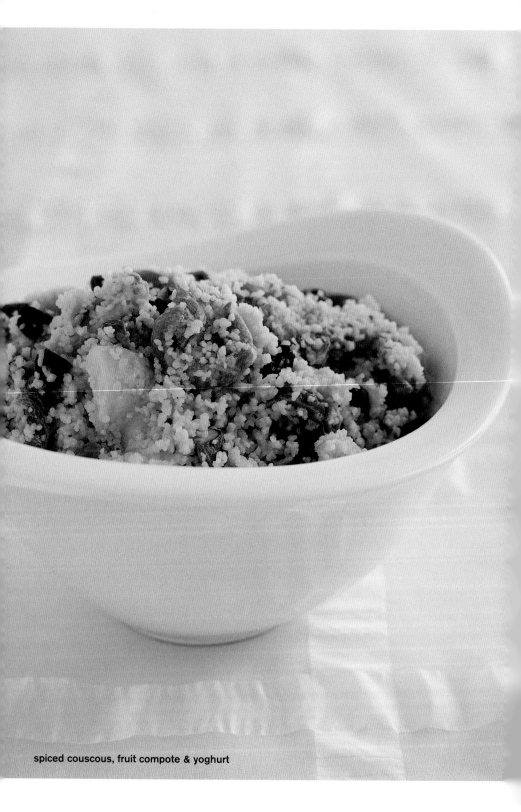

spiced couscous, fruit compote & yoghurt

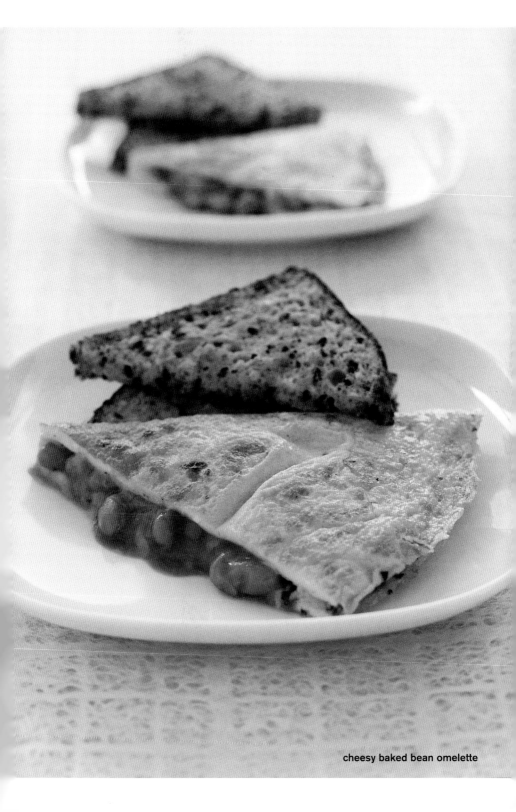

cheesy baked bean omelette

CHEESY BAKED BEAN OMELETTE

4 eggs, lightly beaten

2 tablespoons chopped
fresh parsley

15 g (1/2 oz) reduced-fat
polyunsaturated margarine

200 g (61/2 oz) can reduced-salt
baked beans

1/3 cup (40 g/11/3 oz) grated
reduced-fat cheddar cheese

1 Whisk the eggs and parsley together.

2 Melt the margarine in a 30 cm (12 in) non-stick fry pan. Pour in the egg mixture and swirl to coat the base of the pan.

3 Cook over medium heat for 3 minutes until the sides begin to set, then gently lift the edge and allow the uncooked egg to run underneath.

4 Top with baked beans, evenly spread, and sprinkle with the grated cheese. Cook for 3 minutes or until the underneath just begins to set. Fold in half using an egg slice. Cut into wedges and serve with toasted grainy bread. Serves 4

per serve ǀ fat 9 g ǀ protein 12 g ǀ carbohydrate 6 g ǀ fibre 2.5 g ǀ cholesterol 193.5 mg ǀ energy 635 kj (150 cal) ǀ gi 46 ▼ low

WARM FRUIT SALAD WITH YOGHURT

700 g (1 lb 61/2 oz) peeled
rockmelon, sliced

200 g (61/2 oz) strawberries,
cut into halves

2 kiwifruit, peeled and sliced

500 g (1 lb) peeled pineapple

1/3 cup (80 ml/22/3 fl oz)
passionfruit pulp

1/2 cup (125 ml/4 fl oz)
unsweetened pineapple juice

200 ml (61/2 fl oz) low-fat
plain yoghurt

1 cup (130 g/41/2 oz) natural
muesli

1 Put the rockmelon, strawberries, kiwifruit and pineapple into a bowl and gently mix to combine.

2 Put the passionfruit and pineapple juice into a pan, gently heat until warm and stir to combine.

3 Pour over the fruit salad and gently mix to coat the fruit in the liquid.

4 Spoon fruit salad into wide-topped glasses and top with a spoonful of yoghurt and muesli. Serves 4

per serve ǀ fat 2.5 g ǀ protein 9.5 g ǀ carbohydrate 44 g ǀ fibre 12.5 g ǀ cholesterol 2.5 mg ǀ energy 1025 kj (245 cal) ǀ gi 53 ▼ low

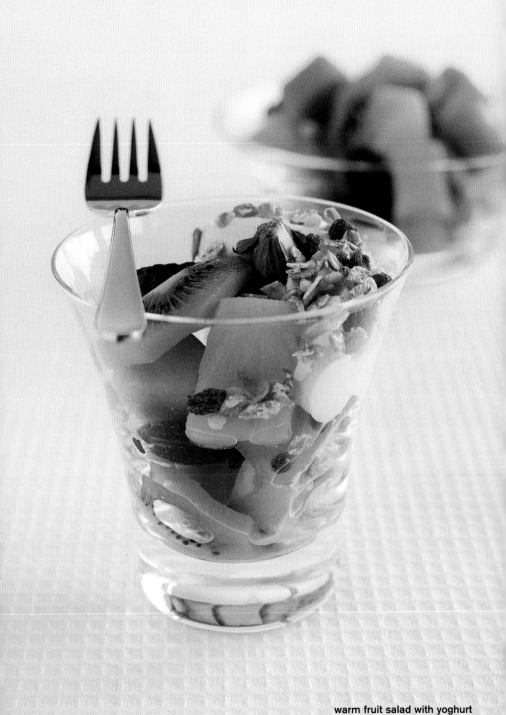

warm fruit salad with yoghurt

SWEET POTATO CAKES WITH ROCKET SALAD

**430 g (15 oz) peeled orange
 sweet potato**
1 egg, lightly beaten
1 tablespoon plain flour
olive oil spray
**4 vine-ripened tomatoes,
 halved lengthwise**
cracked black pepper
50 g (1²/₃ oz) baby rocket (arugula)
**1 avocado, peeled and cut
 into wedges**

1 Preheat oven to 200°C (400°F/Gas 6).

2 Coarsely grate the sweet potato into a bowl, squeeze out any excess moisture and discard it.

3 Add the egg and flour to the sweet potato and mix gently to combine.

4 Shape 2 tablespoons of the mixture into 8 balls and flatten slightly to make evenly-sized potato cakes. Arrange in a non-stick baking tray, spray lightly with olive oil spray, and bake for 25-30 minutes or until cooked through.

5 Put the tomatoes onto a non-stick baking tray, sprinkle with cracked black pepper and bake at the same time as the potato cakes for 30 minutes or until they are soft.

6 Divide potato cakes among 4 plates and serve with tomatoes, rocket and avocado. Serves 4

per serve ╎ fat 13.5 g ╎ protein 7 g ╎ carbohydrate 21 g ╎ fibre 3 g ╎ cholesterol 47 mg ╎ energy 980 kj (235 cal) ╎ gi 52 ▼ low

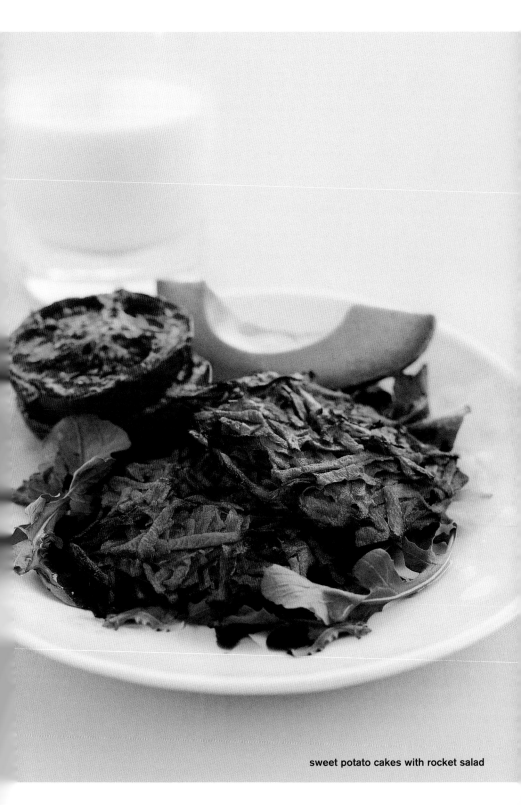

sweet potato cakes with rocket salad

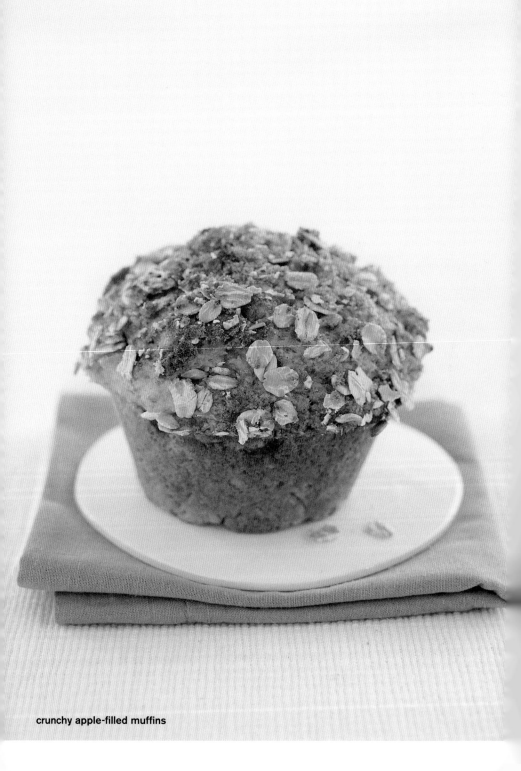

crunchy apple-filled muffins

CRUNCHY APPLE-FILLED MUFFINS

1 Preheat oven to 190°C (375°F/Gas 5). Lightly spray a 6 x ½ cup (125 ml/4 fl oz) capacity non-stick muffin pan with canola oil spray.
2 Sift the flours and cinnamon into a bowl, stir in the brown sugar or sweetener, and make a well in the center. Whisk together the egg, buttermilk and oil, pour into the well and fold in gently until just combined.
3 Half-fill each muffin hole using half the total mixture, top with a spoonful of pie apple, then fill each muffin hole with the remaining mixture.
4 Sprinkle the combined rolled oats and sugar over the top and bake for 20 minutes, or until the muffins are risen and start to come away from the side of the pan. Allow to cool for a couple of minutes before turning out on a wire rack to cool. Makes 6

per muffin (sugar) | fat 9 g | protein 8 g | carbohydrate 47 g | fibre 4.5 g | cholesterol 35 mg | energy 1245 kj (295 cal) | gi 62 ◆ med
per muffin (sweetener) | fat 9 g | protein 8 g | carbohydrate 38 g | fibre 4.5 g | cholesterol 35 mg | energy 1105 kj (265 cal) | gi 60 ◆ med

canola oil spray
1 cup (150 g/5 oz) wholemeal
self-raising flour
1 cup (125 g/4 oz)
self-raising flour
1 teaspoon ground cinnamon
¼ cup (60 g/2 oz) brown sugar
or low-calorie sweetener
suitable for cooking
1 egg, lightly beaten
1 cup (250 ml/8 fl oz) buttermilk
2 tablespoons vegetable oil
200 g (6½ oz) can pie apple
2 tablespoons raw rolled oats
1 tablespoon brown sugar

FILO FRUIT & NUT SHEETS WITH SPICED MILK

4 sheets filo (phyllo) pastry

100 g (3¹/₃ oz) sultanas

¹/₂ cup (55 g/1²/₃ oz) walnuts,
   roughly chopped

¹/₄ cup (30 g/1 oz) flaked almonds

4 cups (1 litre/32 fl oz) skim
   or no-fat milk

¹/₂ teaspoon ground cinnamon

1 Preheat oven to 200°C (400°F/Gas 6).

2 Lay the filo sheets out flat in single layers on 2 non-stick baking trays. Bake for about 15 minutes or until crisp and golden. Break the sheets into large pieces.

3 Arrange a layer of cooked filo into 4 individual cereal bowls, top with some sultanas, walnuts and almonds, top with more pastry and finish with the remaining sultanas and nuts.

4 Heat the milk and cinnamon in a pan just until it comes to the boil. Pour the hot milk over the layered fruit and filo and serve immediately. Serves 4

per serve | **fat 13.5 g** | **protein 14.5 g** | **carbohydrate 40.5 g** | **fibre 3 g** | **cholesterol 18 mg** | **energy 1410 kj (335 cal)** | **gi 48** ▼ **low**

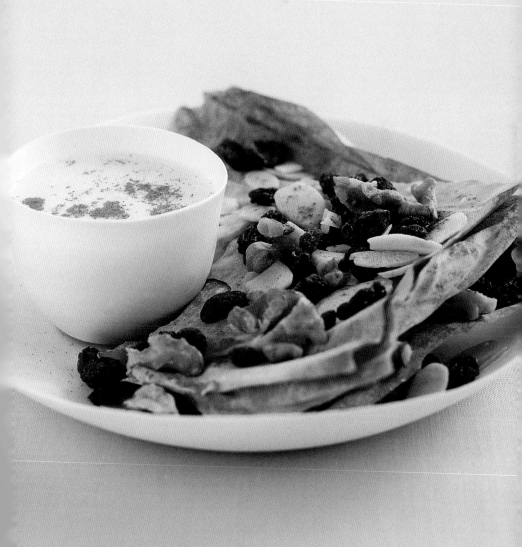

filo fruit & nut sheets with spiced milk

SOUPS & SNACKS

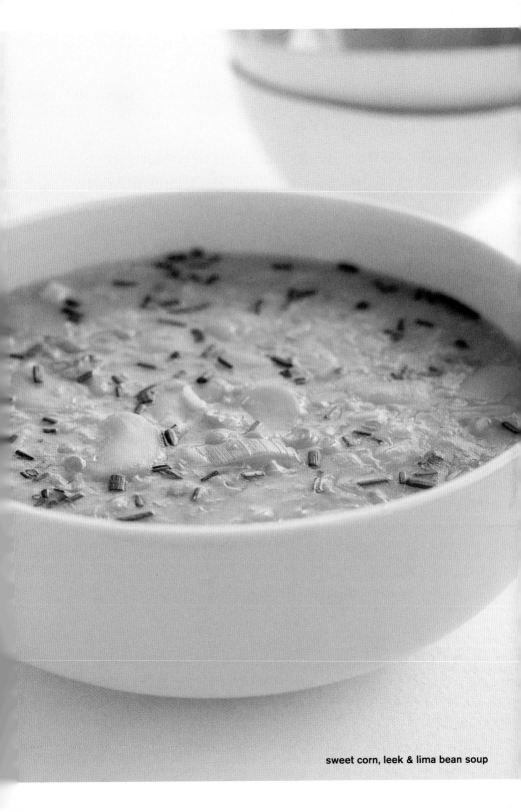

sweet corn, leek & lima bean soup

SWEET CORN, LEEK & LIMA BEAN SOUP

200 g (6½ oz) dried lima beans,
  soaked in cold water overnight
2 teaspoons olive oil
1 medium leek, sliced
840 g (1 lb 11 oz) can
  creamed corn
1 cup (200 g/6½ oz) fresh
  or frozen corn kernels
5 cups (1.25 litres/40 fl oz)
  reduced-salt chicken stock
⅓ cup (70 g/2⅓ oz) basmati rice
2 tablespoons snipped
  fresh chives

1 Rinse the lima beans under cold water. Simmer in a large pan of water for 40 minutes or until soft. Drain and remove any loose skins.

2 Heat the oil in a large pan, add the leek and cook over medium heat for 5 minutes or until soft.

3 Add all the corn, stock and rice. Bring to the boil, reduce heat and simmer, stirring occasionally, for 25 minutes or until the corn and rice are soft.

4 Add the beans and chives to the soup and cook until warmed through. Serve hot. Serves 6

per serve | fat 4.5 g | protein 14.5 g | carbohydrate 52.5 g | fibre 12.5 g | cholesterol 0 mg | energy 1300 kj (310 cal) | gi 45 ▼ low

SIMPLE CHICKEN NOODLE SOUP

100 g (3⅓ oz) mung bean
  (glass) noodles
6 cups (1.5 litres/48 fl oz)
  reduced-salt chicken stock
1 tablespoon reduced-salt
  soy sauce
2 (600 g/1 lb 3 oz) medium
  chicken breasts, skinless
100 g (3⅓ oz) snowpeas, sliced
200 g (6½ oz) broccoli florets
1 cup (150 g/5 oz) peas

1 Put noodles into a bowl, cover with boiling water and set aside for 10 minutes or until soft. Drain well.

2 Put the stock and soy into a large fry pan, bring to the boil and reduce heat to a simmer.

3 Add the chicken breasts, cover and cook for 10-15 minutes or until the chicken is tender and its juices run clear when tested with a knife. Remove and allow to cool slightly.

4 Finely shred the chicken and return to the stock.

5 Add the snowpeas, broccoli and peas and cook for 5 minutes or until the vegetables are soft.

6 Divide the noodles evenly among the bowls and ladle soup over the top. Serves 6

per serve | fat 6.5 g | protein 27 g | carbohydrate 19.5 g | fibre 3 g | cholesterol 63 mg | energy 1030 kj (245 cal) | gi 39 ▼ low

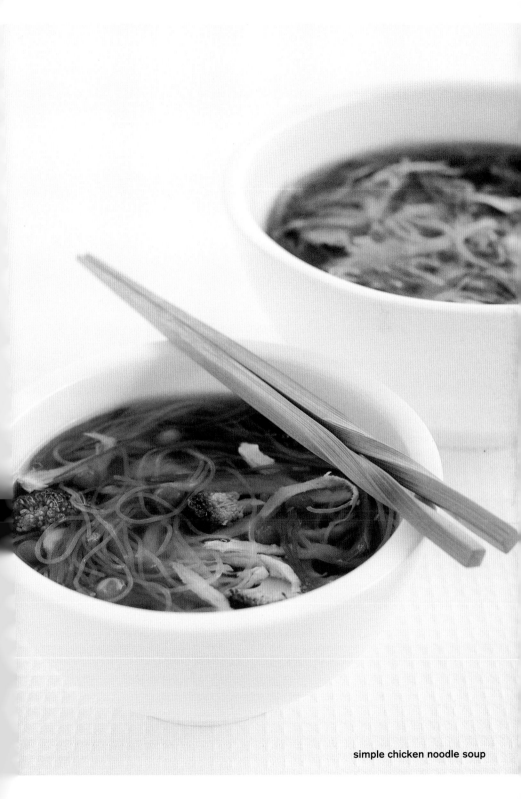

simple chicken noodle soup

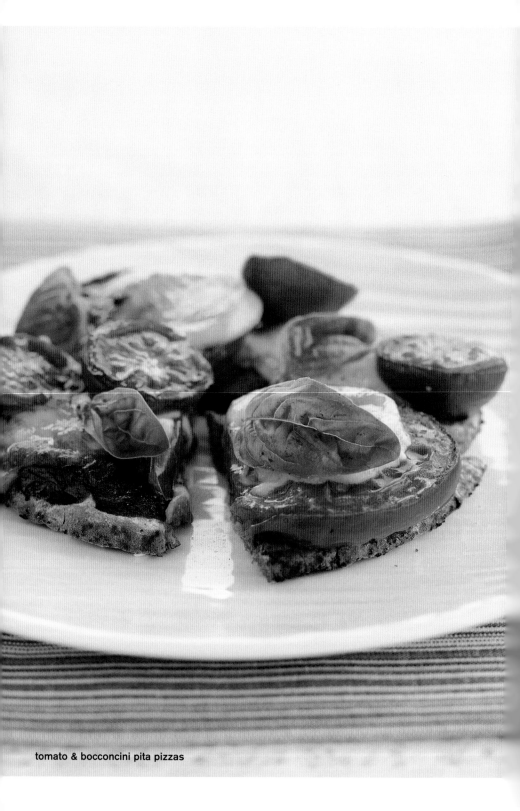

tomato & bocconcini pita pizzas

TOMATO & BOCCONCINI PITA PIZZAS

1 Preheat oven to 220°C (425°F/Gas 7).

2 Spread the tomato paste over the pita.
Layer the bocconcini and both types of tomato
over the paste and drizzle the balsamic evenly.

3 Bake for 10-15 minutes or until the base
is crisp and the bocconcini is golden.

4 Scatter the basil leaves over the top
before serving. Serves 4 as a snack

per serve | **fat 4.5 g** | **protein 10.5 g** | **carbohydrate
37 g** | **fibre 7 g** | **cholesterol 6.5 mg** | **energy 980 kj
(235 cal)** | **gi 55** ▼ **low**

2 tablespoons tomato paste

4 (280 g/9 oz) medium
  wholemeal pita bread

75 g (2½ oz) bocconcini
  (small, fresh mozzarella
  cheese), thinly sliced

2 (250 g/8 oz) vine-ripened
  tomatoes, cut into thick slices

200 g (6½ oz) cherry
  tomatoes, halved

2 teaspoons balsamic vinegar

2 tablespoons torn fresh
  basil leaves

ROAST GARLIC & BEAN DIP WITH PITA CRISPS

1 Preheat oven to 180°C (350°F/Gas 4).

2 Put the garlic into a baking dish and bake
for 30 minutes or until soft. Remove and discard
the skin and set the flesh aside.

3 Cut the pita into triangles, spray lightly with olive
oil spray and sprinkle with cumin seeds. Bake on
a non-stick baking tray for 15 minutes or until crisp.

4 While the pita crisps bake, put the garlic flesh,
beans and cream cheese into a food processor
and process until creamy. Sprinkle the dip with
paprika and serve with pita. Serves 8 as a snack

per serve | **fat 6.5 g** | **protein 6 g** | **carbohydrate 15 g**
| **fibre 3 g** | **cholesterol 15.5 mg** | **energy 590 kj
(140 cal)** | **gi 51** ▼ **low**

1 head garlic, kept whole
  and skin on

3 (210 g/6¾ oz) wholemeal
  pita bread

olive oil spray

1 tablespoon cumin seeds

400 g (13 oz) can butter beans,
  drained weight 300 g (10 oz)

250 g (8 oz) light cream cheese

¼ teaspoon paprika

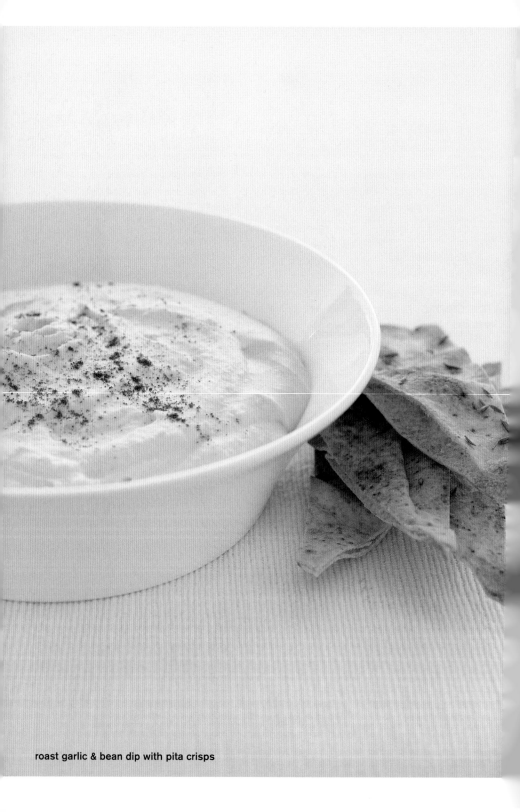

roast garlic & bean dip with pita crisps

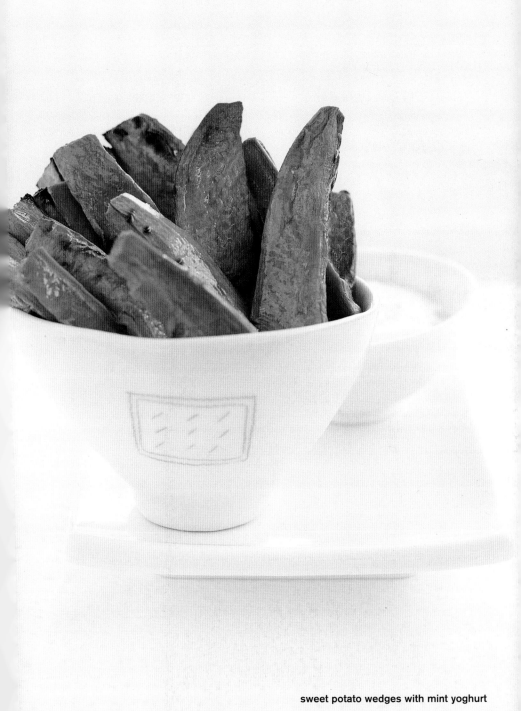

sweet potato wedges with mint yoghurt

SWEET POTATO WEDGES WITH MINT YOGHURT

750 g (1½ lb) peeled orange
   sweet potato
olive oil spray
¼ teaspoon ground cumin
200 ml (6½ fl oz) no-fat
   plain yoghurt
1 clove garlic, crushed
2 tablespoons finely shredded
   fresh mint

1 Preheat oven to 220°C (425°F/Gas 7).
2 Cut the sweet potato into long, thick wedges and lightly spray with olive oil spray. Put onto a non-stick baking tray and bake for 40 minutes or until tender.
3 Put the cumin, yoghurt, garlic and mint into a bowl and mix to combine. Serve wedges with yoghurt dip on the side. Serves 4 as a snack

per serve | **fat 1.5 g** | **protein 6.5 g** | **carbohydrate 29.5 g** | **fibre 3.5 g** | **cholesterol 2.5 mg** | **energy 675 kj (160 cal)** | **gi 51** ▼ **low**

SWEET CORN WITH SESAME HERB CRUST

4 (300 g/10 oz) cobs sweet corn
15 g (½ oz) reduced-fat
   polyunsaturated margarine
1 clove garlic, crushed
1 tablespoon chopped
   fresh parsley
2 tablespoons ready-made
   sesame seed mix

1 Cook the sweet corn in a large pan of boiling water for 10 minutes or until the kernels are tender. Drain and set aside.
2 Put the margarine, garlic and parsley into a bowl and mix to combine. Spread the mixture evenly down the sides of the corn cobs.
3 Roll the cobs in the seed mix until coated. Serve hot. Serves 4 as a snack

per serve | **fat 6 g** | **protein 4 g** | **carbohydrate 15.5 g** | **fibre 3 g** | **cholesterol 0 mg** | **energy 555 kj (130 cal)** | **gi 48** ▼ **low**

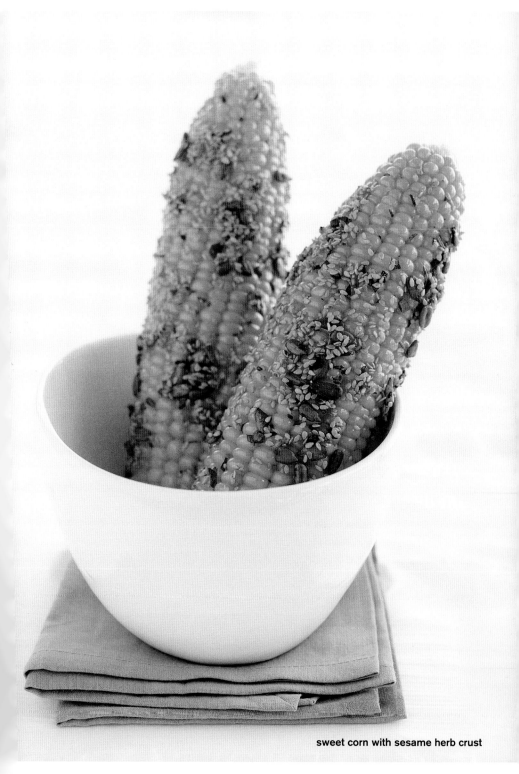

sweet corn with sesame herb crust

ITALIAN VEGETABLE, BEAN & PASTA SOUP

2 teaspoons olive oil

1 medium onion,
coarsely chopped

2 cloves garlic, crushed

1 small eggplant (aubergine),
coarsely chopped

2 medium red capsicums
(bell peppers), seeded
and coarsely chopped

1 medium green capsicum
(bell pepper), seeded
and coarsely chopped

2 medium zucchini
(courgette), thickly sliced

800 g (1 lb 10 oz) can
chopped tomatoes

1 bay leaf

1 teaspoon dried Italian
mixed herbs

5 cups (1.25 litres/40 fl oz)
reduced-salt vegetable stock

400 g (13 oz) can butter beans,
drained weight 300 g (10 oz)

1 cup (155 g/5 oz) frozen broad
beans, defrosted and peeled

100 g (3⅓ oz) fettuccine, broken

1 Heat the oil in a large pan, add the onion and cook over medium heat for 5 minutes or until the onion is golden.

2 Add the garlic and eggplant and cook for 5 minutes or until the eggplant is golden.

3 Add the capsicum and zucchini and cook for 5 minutes or until just tender. Stir in the tomatoes, bay leaf, mixed herbs and stock. Bring to the boil, reduce heat and simmer for 15 minutes or until the vegetables are tender.

4 Add the butter beans, broad beans and fettuccine and cook for 5 minutes, stirring occasionally, or until the fettuccine is al dente (cooked, but still with a bite to it). Serves 6

per serve | **fat 3 g** | **protein 9.5 g** | **carbohydrate 22 g** | **fibre 6.5 g** | **cholesterol 0 mg** | **energy 665 kj (160 cal)** | **gi 38** ▼ **low**

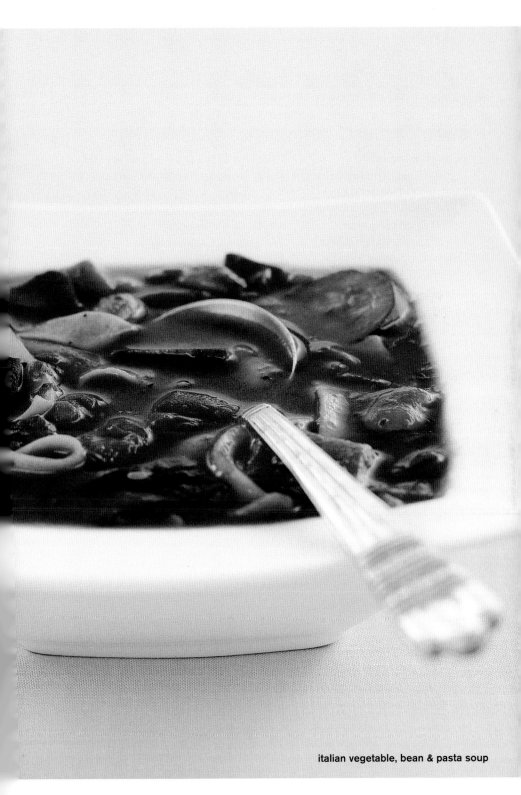

italian vegetable, bean & pasta soup

SWEET POTATO, GINGER & SOYBEAN SOUP

2 teaspoons sesame oil

1 medium onion, finely chopped

1 tablespoon finely grated
   fresh ginger

500 g (1 lb) peeled orange
   sweet potato, cut into chunks

1 tablespoon reduced-salt
   soy sauce

5 cups (1.25 litres/40 fl oz)
   reduced-salt vegetable stock

2 star anise

1 cup (15 g/½ oz) dried
   Chinese mushrooms, halved

300 g (10 oz) can soybeans,
   drained weight 220 g (7 oz)

1 bunch (200 g/6½ oz) broccolini
   or broccoli, roughly chopped

2 tablespoons chopped fresh
   coriander (cilantro)

1 Heat the oil in a large pan, add the onion and ginger and cook over medium heat for 3 minutes or until the onion is golden.

2 Add the sweet potato and cook for 5 minutes or until it starts to soften.

3 Add the soy, stock, star anise, Chinese mushrooms and soybeans. Bring to the boil, reduce heat, cover and simmer for 30 minutes or until the sweet potato is soft.

4 Stir in the broccolini and coriander, simmer for 3 minutes uncovered or just until the greens wilt. Serve hot. Serves 4

per serve | fat **7 g** | protein **14 g** | carbohydrate **24.5 g** | fibre **6 g** | cholesterol **0 mg** | energy **890 kj (215 cal)** | gi **41** ▼ low

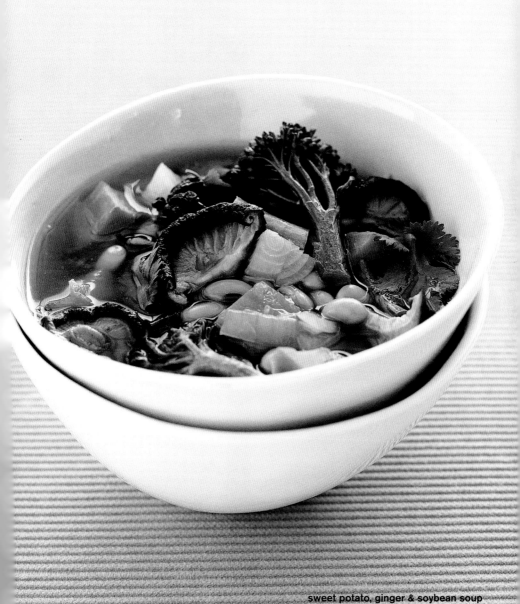

sweet potato, ginger & soybean soup

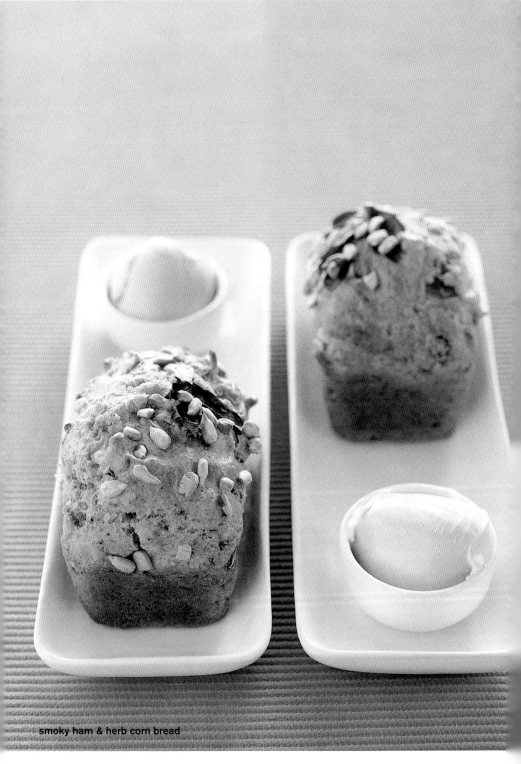

smoky ham & herb corn bread

SMOKY HAM & HERB CORN BREAD

1 Preheat oven to 180°C (350°F/Gas 4).
Lightly grease a 23 cm x 8 cm (9 in x 3 in)
loaf tin or 8 individual serve sized mini loaf tins.
2 Sift the flour, baking powder and paprika into
a bowl. Add the cornmeal, cheese, ham, herbs,
eggs, soy milk and oil and mix to combine.
3 Spoon the mixture into the prepared tin and
decorate with parsley and sunflower seeds.
4 Bake for 45 minutes for the large loaf or 20
minutes for the mini loaves.
5 Allow to cool in the tin for 5 minutes before
turning out on a wire rack to cool completely.
6 Serve warm with reduced-fat polyunsaturated
margarine. Serves 8 as a snack

per serve | fat 9.5 g | protein 10.5 g | carbohydrate
25.5 g | fibre 1.5 g | cholesterol 56 mg | energy 965 kj
(230 cal) | gi 65 ◆ med

1 cup (150 g/5 oz)
self-raising flour
2 teaspoons baking powder
1 teaspoon sweet paprika
3/4 cup (110 g/3 1/2 oz)
fine cornmeal (polenta)
1/3 cup (40 g/1 1/3 oz) grated
reduced-fat cheddar cheese
100 g (3 1/3 oz) 97% fat-free
smoked ham, chopped
1/3 cup (10 g/1/3 oz) chopped
fresh herbs
2 eggs, lightly beaten
1 cup (250 ml/8 fl oz) reduced-fat
soy milk
2 tablespoons canola oil
extra fresh parsley leaves,
to decorate
2 tablespoons sunflower seeds

DRIED APRICOT & PEACH CEREAL BARS

200 g (6½ oz) dried apricots

200 g (6½ oz) dried peaches

3 cups (285 g/9 oz) raw
  rolled oats

⅓ cup (40 g/1⅓ oz) plain flour

2 eggs, lightly beaten

60 g (2 oz) reduced-fat
  polyunsaturated margarine

75 g (2½ oz) milk cooking
  chocolate, chopped

1 Preheat oven to 180°C (350°F/Gas 4).

2 Lightly grease and line a 18 cm x 28 cm
(7 in x 11 in) shallow baking tin.

3 Put the apricots and peaches into a food
processor and pulse until finely chopped, or
alternatively chop finely with a sharp knife.

4 Put the dried fruit, rolled oats, flour, eggs
and melted margarine into a bowl and mix well.

5 Press mixture into the prepared tin and bake
for 15-20 minutes or until firm. Cool in the tin.

6 Put the chocolate into a small heatproof
bowl over a small pan of gently simmering water.
Do not let any water come into contact with
the chocolate or it will be ruined.

7 Drizzle the melted chocolate over the slice
and allow to set. Use a serrated knife to cut
the slice into even bars. Makes 18

per bar | **fat 5 g** | **protein 4 g** | **carbohydrate 23.5 g**
| **fibre 3 g** | **cholesterol 21.5 mg** | **energy 645 kj**
(155 cal) | **gi 40** ▼ **low**

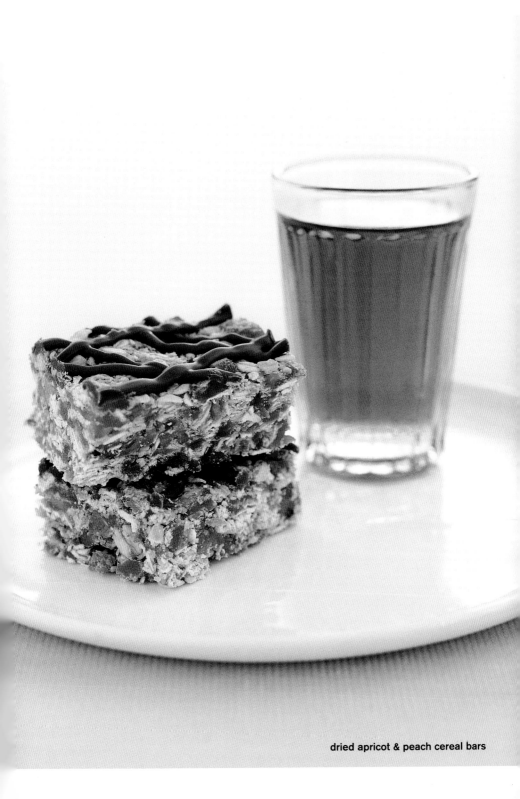

dried apricot & peach cereal bars

LUNCH

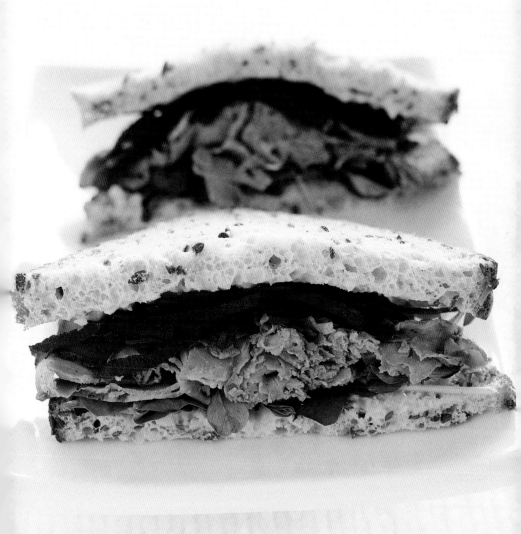

roast beef & horseradish sandwiches

ROAST BEEF & HORSERADISH SANDWICHES

8 slices (320 g/10²/₃ oz) grainy
  soy and linseed bread
2 tablespoons bottled
  horseradish cream
250 g (8 oz) lean roast beef,
  thinly sliced
100 g (3¹/₃ oz) beetroot,
  peeled and grated
50 g (1²/₃ oz) snowpea sprouts
cracked black pepper

1 Spread 4 slices of bread with horseradish.
2 Top with the shaved beef, grated beetroot and
snowpea sprouts. Sprinkle with cracked black
pepper. Top with the remaining bread slices,
cut and serve. Serves 4

**per serve | fat 6 g | protein 23.5 g | carbohydrate
33.5 g | fibre 4 g | cholesterol 44.5 mg | energy
1190 kj (285 cal) | gi 34 ▼ low**

PRAWN SUSHI NESTS

1 cup (200 g/6¹/₂ oz) Japanese
  short-grain rice
1 tablespoon Japanese
  rice vinegar
10 (50 g/1²/₃ oz) sheets
  nori seaweed, cut in half
1 avocado, peeled and chopped
350 g (12 oz) cooked medium
  king prawns (20), peeled
  but with tails left on
1 medium Lebanese cucumber,
  unpeeled and thinly sliced
1 tablespoon pickled ginger,
  finely chopped
wasabi (Japanese horseradish),
  to serve
reduced-salt soy sauce, to serve

1 Put the rice into a pan and add 3 cups
(750 ml/24 fl oz) cold water. Bring to the boil
and cook over medium heat for 5 minutes or
until tunnels appear on the surface of the rice.
2 Reduce the heat to low, cover and cook for
10 minutes or until the rice is soft. Remove from
heat, stir in the vinegar and set aside to cool.
3 Line 10 x ¹/₃ cup (80 ml/2²/₃ fl oz) capacity
non-stick muffin holes with double thickness
nori, spoon 2 tablespoons of rice into each of
the holes, then top each equally with avocado,
prawns, cucumber and ginger.
4 Lift the nests out gently and serve
immediately with wasabi and soy. Makes 10

**per nest | fat 5 g | protein 10 g | carbohydrate 17 g
| fibre 3 g | cholesterol 57 mg | energy 645 kj
(155 cal) | gi 47 ▼ low**

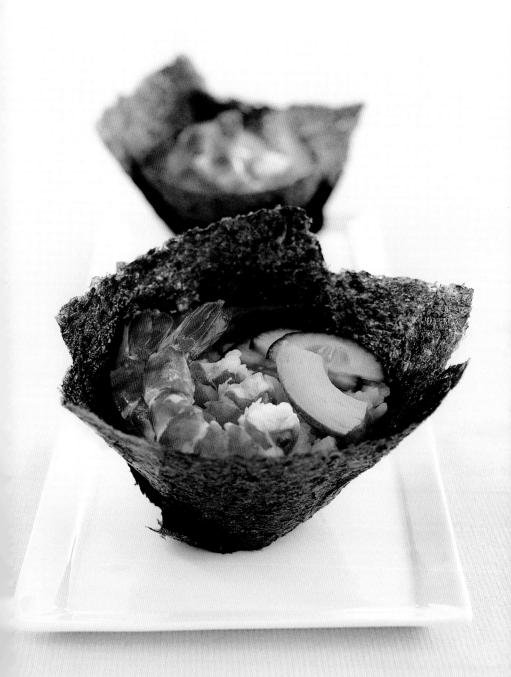

prawn sushi nests

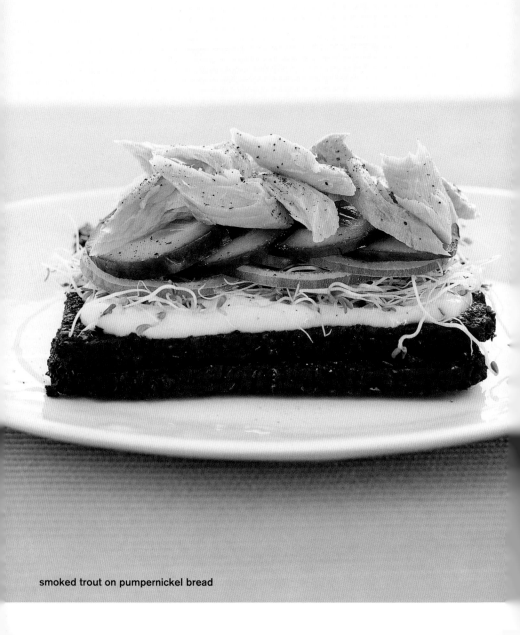

smoked trout on pumpernickel bread

SMOKED TROUT ON PUMPERNICKEL BREAD

1 Cut the cucumber and onion into paper-thin slices. Put them into a non-metallic bowl, pour over the vinegar, mix and allow to stand for 10 minutes.
2 Spread the bread with the mayonnaise and top evenly with the sprouts, cucumber and onion.
3 Break trout into large flakes, arrange on top of the cucumber and sprinkle with black pepper. Serves 4

per serve | fat 6.5 g | protein 26.5 g | carbohydrate 49 g | fibre 10 g | cholesterol 55 mg | energy 1525 kj (365 cal) | gi 47 ▼ low

2 Lebanese cucumbers, unpeeled
1 medium red (Spanish) onion
2 tablespoons apple cider vinegar
8 slices (400 g/13 oz)
    pumpernickel bread
2 tablespoons low-fat mayonnaise
1 cup (60 g/2 oz) alfalfa sprouts
1 smoked rainbow trout,
    skin and bones removed
    (300 g/10 oz trimmed weight)
cracked black pepper

MEXICAN MEATLOAF

1 Preheat oven to 180°C (350°F/Gas 4). Grease and line the base of a 20 cm x 10 cm (8 in x 4 in) loaf tin.
2 Put the mince, cumin, paprika, breadcrumbs, onion, carrot, egg and kidney beans into a bowl and mix to combine.
3 Press the mixture into the prepared tin. Spread the tomato salsa over the top and bake for 45 minutes or until cooked through. Drain off any excess moisture.
4 Serve slices with a leafy green salad. Serves 8

per serve | fat 9 g | protein 30 g | carbohydrate 13.5 g | fibre 3.5 g | cholesterol 119 mg | energy 1075 kj (255 cal) | gi 47 ▼ low

1 kg (2 lb) lean chicken mince
1/2 teaspoon ground cumin
1/2 teaspoon paprika
70 g (2 1/3 oz) fresh wholegrain
    breadcrumbs
1 medium onion, grated
1 medium carrot, grated
1 egg, lightly beaten
400 g (13 oz) can red kidney
    beans, drained weight
    300 g (10 oz)
1/2 cup (135 g/4 1/2 oz) medium
    heat, bottled tomato salsa

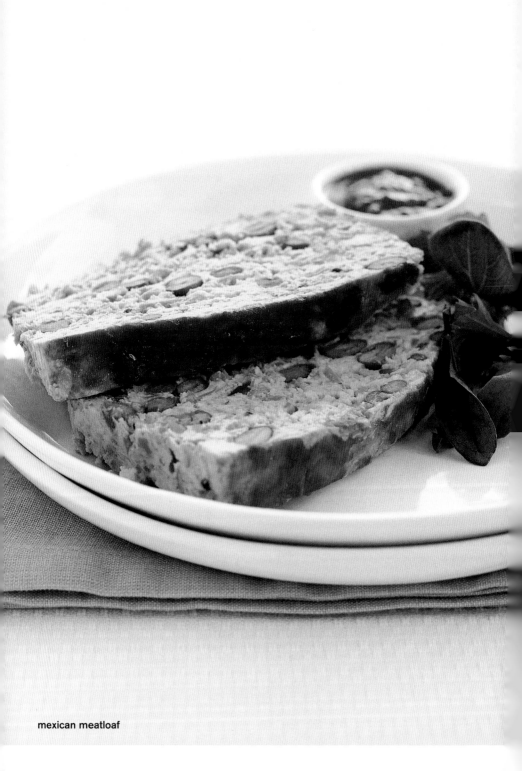

mexican meatloaf

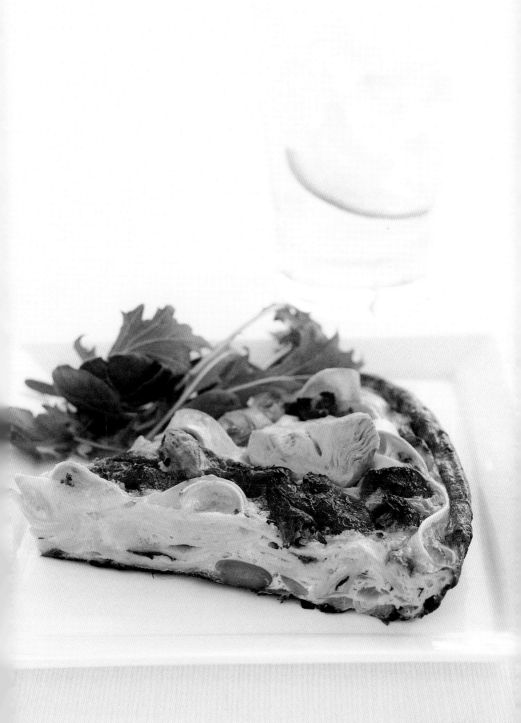

antipasto frittata

ANTIPASTO FRITTATA

100 g (3⅓ oz) fettuccine
2 teaspoons olive oil
1 medium onion, thinly sliced
1 cup (150 g/5 oz) fresh or
  frozen broad beans, peeled
6 eggs, lightly beaten
½ cup (125 ml/4 fl oz) skim or
  no-fat milk
2 tablespoons chopped fresh basil
⅓ cup (30 g/1 oz) grated
  parmesan cheese
150 g (5 oz) canned artichoke
  hearts in brine, drained
  and quartered
100 g (3⅓ oz) semi-dried
  tomatoes

1 Cook the fettuccine in a large pan of rapidly boiling water until al dente (cooked, but still with a bite to it). Drain well and set aside.

2 Heat the oil in a 30 cm (12 in) non-stick fry pan, add the onion and broad beans and cook over medium heat until the onion is golden.

3 Whisk together the eggs, milk, basil and parmesan and pour into the pan. Arrange the fettuccine, artichokes and tomatoes evenly in the pan. Cook over a low-medium heat for about 10 minutes or until the edges of the egg mixture start to set.

4 Transfer to a preheated grill and cook under a medium heat for 5-10 minutes or until the center of the egg mixture is just set.

5 Allow to cool for 5 minutes before sliding the frittata out and cutting into wedges. Serve hot or cold with a mixed green salad. Serves 6

per serve ⏐ fat 9 g ⏐ protein 15.5 g ⏐ carbohydrate 20.5 g ⏐ fibre 5.5 g ⏐ cholesterol 195.5 mg ⏐ energy 950 kj (225 cal) ⏐ gi 35 ▼ low

QUICK FRIED RICE

1 tablespoon vegetable oil
4 spring onions (scallions), sliced
2 eggs, lightly beaten
125 g (4 oz) 97% fat-free ham,
  thinly sliced
4 cups (760 g/1½ lb) cooked,
  cold basmati rice
1 cup (200 g/6½ oz) fresh or
  frozen corn kernels
1 cup (150 g/5 oz) peas
1 tablespoon reduced-salt
  soy sauce

1 Heat the oil in a wok, add the spring onions and stir fry over medium heat for 2 minutes or until soft.

2 Add the eggs and stir gently for 1-2 minutes or just until the eggs begin to scramble.

3 Add the ham and rice and stir fry for 3 minutes. Stir in the corn, peas and soy and heat through. Serve hot or cold. Serves 6

Note: 1¼ cups (250 g/8 oz) of uncooked basmati rice yields 4 cups cooked rice.

per serve ⏐ fat 6.5 g ⏐ protein 12 g ⏐ carbohydrate 44 g ⏐ fibre 3.5 g ⏐ cholesterol 73.5 mg ⏐ energy 1185 kj (285 cal) ⏐ gi 56 ◆ med

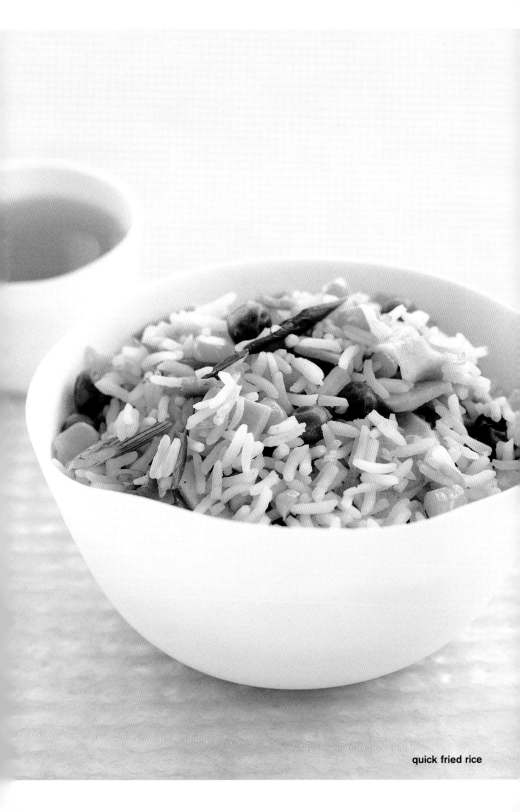

quick fried rice

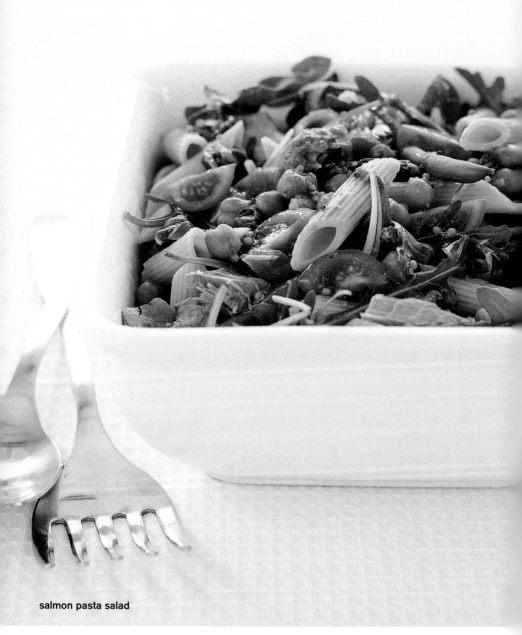

salmon pasta salad

SALMON PASTA SALAD

1 Cook the pasta in a large pan of rapidly boiling water until al dente (cooked, but still with a bite to it). Rinse under cold water and drain well.
2 Steam the green beans until tender.
3 Break the salmon into large chunks and mix gently together with the pasta, beans, chickpeas, quartered tomatoes, sliced onion, rocket and capers.
4 Whisk together the mustard, vinegar, orange juice and olive oil. Pour the dressing over the salad and mix through. Serves 6

per serve | fat 8 g | protein 22.5 g | carbohydrate 45 g | fibre 6 g | cholesterol 44 mg | energy 1455 kj (345 cal) | gi 42 ▼ low

300 g (10 oz) penne pasta
200 g (6½ oz) trimmed green beans
425 g (14 oz) can pink salmon
  in water with no added salt
400 g (13 oz) can chickpeas,
  drained weight 300 g (10 oz)
250 g (8 oz) cherry tomatoes
1 medium red (Spanish) onion
50 g (1¾ oz) rocket (arugula)
2 tablespoons chopped capers
3 teaspoons wholegrain mustard
2 tablespoons balsamic vinegar
¼ cup (60 ml/2 fl oz)
  unsweetened orange juice
1 tablespoon olive oil

THAI CHICKEN & GREEN HERB SALAD

1 Put noodles into a bowl, cover with boiling water and set aside for 10 minutes or until soft. Drain well.
2 Put the chicken breasts into a deep fry pan, cover with water and simmer over low heat for 20 minutes or until tender. Allow to cool slightly, then remove from the liquid and shred finely.
3 Cook the beans and snowpeas in boiling water for 2-3 minutes or until bright green and just tender. Drain and rinse in cold water.
4 Put the noodles, chicken, beans, snowpeas, spring onions, cucumber, cabbage and mint into a bowl and toss to combine.
5 Whisk together the lime juice, apple juice, oyster sauce and sesame oil and pour over the salad. Toss together and serve. Serves 6

per serve | fat 6 g | protein 22.5 g | carbohydrate 19 g | fibre 2 g | cholesterol 63 mg | energy 940 kj (225 cal) | gi 38 ▼ low

100 g (3⅓ oz) mung bean
  (glass) noodles
2 (600 g/1 lb 3 oz) medium lean
  chicken breasts, trimmed
  of skin and any visible fat
200 g (6½oz) green beans, trimmed
100 g (3⅓ oz) snowpeas,
  thinly sliced
3 spring onions (scallions), chopped
1 medium cucumber, thinly sliced
2 cups (75 g/2½ oz) Chinese
  cabbage, finely shredded
1cup (20 g/¾ oz) fresh mint leaves
3 tablespoons lime juice
¼ cup (60 ml/2 fl oz)
  unsweetened apple juice
1 tablespoon oyster sauce
1 teaspoon sesame oil

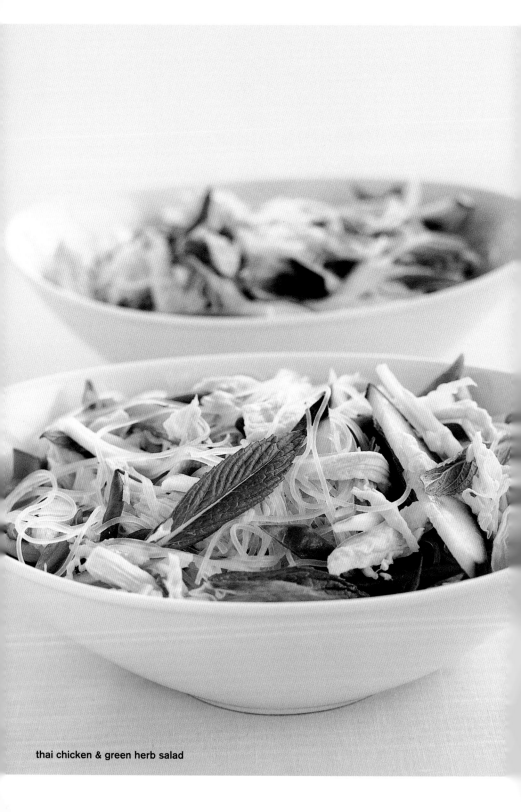

thai chicken & green herb salad

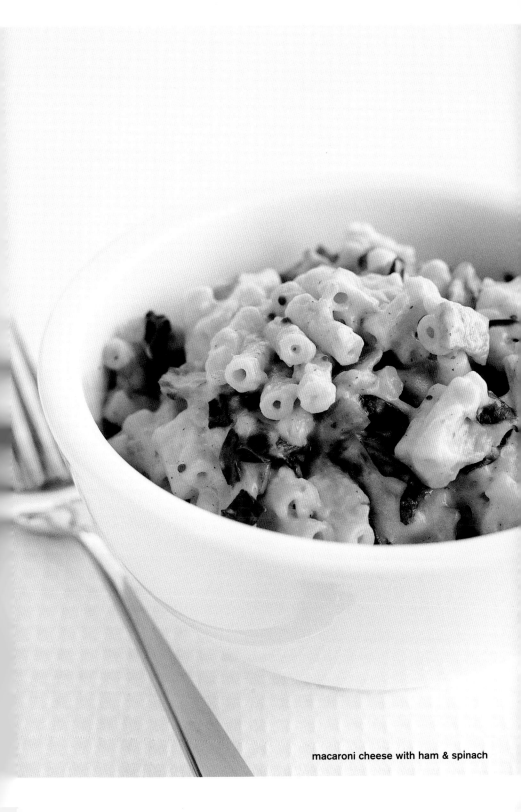

macaroni cheese with ham & spinach

MACARONI CHEESE WITH HAM & SPINACH

200 g (6½ oz) macaroni

30 g (1 oz) reduced-fat
   polyunsaturated margarine

125 g (4 oz) 97% fat-free ham,
   finely sliced

1½ tablespoons plain flour

1¾ cups (440 ml/14 fl oz) skim
   or no-fat milk

1 teaspoon wholegrain mustard

50 g (1⅔ oz) baby spinach,
   roughly chopped

⅓ cup (40 g/1⅓ oz) grated
   reduced-fat cheddar cheese

sea salt

cracked black pepper

1 Cook the pasta in a large pan of rapidly boiling water until al dente (cooked, but still with a bite to it). Drain well and keep warm.

2 Heat the margarine in a fry pan, add the ham and cook over medium-high heat for about 5 minutes or until browned.

3 Stir in the flour and cook, stirring continuously, for 1 minute. Remove the pan from the heat and gradually whisk in the milk. Return to the heat and cook, stirring constantly, for about 2 minutes or until the sauce boils and thickens.

4 Stir in the mustard, spinach and cheese and season to taste with sea salt and pepper. Cook just until the cheese melts.

5 Add the pasta to the pan and stir to coat the pasta with the sauce. Serve immediately. Serves 4

per serve | fat 8 g | protein 19.5 g | carbohydrate 43 g | fibre 2 g | cholesterol 25 mg | energy 1350 kj (320 cal) | gi 46 ▼ low

CHARGRILLED VEGETABLE & RICOTTA SALAD

300 g (10 oz) peeled orange
   sweet potato

2 medium red capsicums (bell
   peppers), cut into thick strips

2 medium zucchini (courgette)

200 g (6½ oz) field mushrooms

1 cup (250 ml/8 fl oz) no-oil,
   no-sugar plain salad dressing

8 slices (240 g/7⅔ oz)
   wholegrain bread

100 g (3⅓ oz) baby spinach

100 g (3⅓ oz) reduced-fat
   ricotta cheese, crumbled

40 g (1⅓ oz) sunflower seeds

1 Put the sweet potato, capsicum, zucchini and mushrooms into a bowl and pour over all but 2 tablespoons of salad dressing. Mix thoroughly.

2 Remove the crusts from the bread and brush the slices with remaining dressing.

3 Cook the vegetables and bread on both sides on a preheated chargrill plate until the vegetables are tender and the bread is grilled.

4 Put the vegetables, bread, spinach, ricotta and sunflower seeds into a bowl and toss gently to combine. Serve hot or cold. Serves 4

per serve | fat 9.5 g | protein 15 g | carbohydrate 37 g | fibre 8.5 g | cholesterol 10.5 mg | energy 1245 kj (300 cal) | gi 47 ▼ low

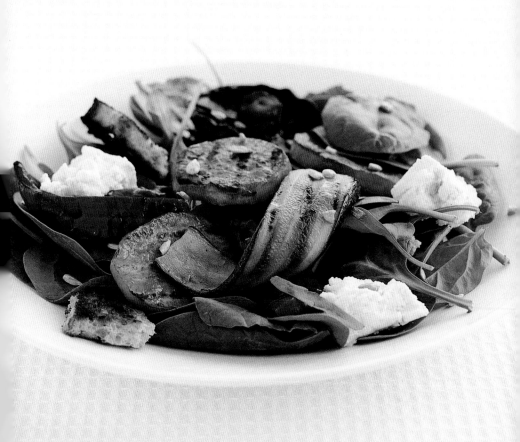

chargrilled vegetable & ricotta salad

DINNER

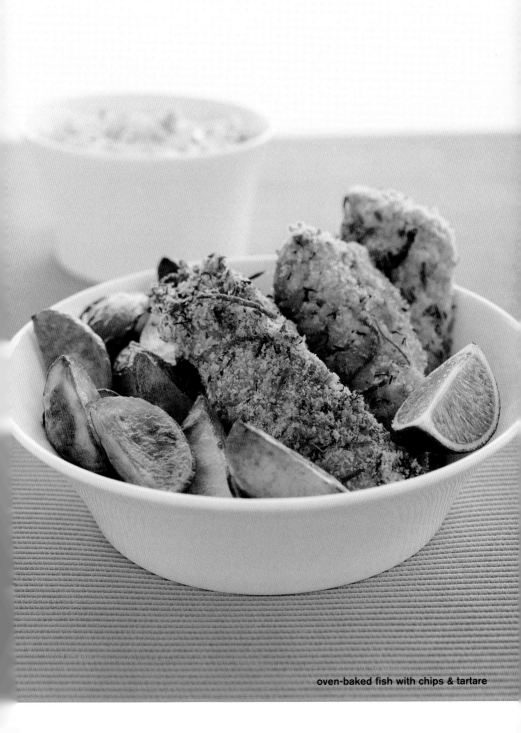

oven-baked fish with chips & tartare

OVEN-BAKED FISH WITH CHIPS & TARTARE

2 tablespoons finely grated
  parmesan cheese
3/4 cup (75 g/2½ oz) dry
  breadcrumbs
1 tablespoon chopped fresh dill
8 (1.25 kg/2½ lb) trimmed,
  firm white fish fillets
1 egg white, lightly beaten
500 g (1 lb) unpeeled baby
  potatoes, cut into thick wedges
olive oil spray
2 tablespoons capers, chopped
3 small gherkins, chopped
2 spring onions (scallions),
  trimmed and chopped
3 tablespoons low-fat mayonnaise
3 tablespoons low-fat
  plain yoghurt
lemon wedges, to serve

1 Preheat oven to 220°C (425°F/Gas 7).
2 Put the parmesan, breadcrumbs and dill onto a flat plate and mix to combine. Dip the fish into the egg white and coat in the crumb mixture.
3 Put the potatoes into a baking dish, spray lightly with olive oil spray and bake for 20 minutes or until the potatoes are golden and tender.
4 Arrange the fish on a separate non-stick baking tray, spray lightly with the olive oil spray and put into the oven with the potatoes for the last 10 minutes of baking. The cooked fish will flake apart easily when tested with the tip of a knife.
5 To make the tartare sauce, put the capers, gherkins, spring onions, mayonnaise and yoghurt into a bowl and mix to combine. Serve the fish and chips with pots of tartare sauce and wedges of lemon. Serves 6

per serve | fat 4.5 g | protein 32.5 g | carbohydrate 24.5 g | fibre 2.5 g | cholesterol 77 mg | energy 1140 kj (270 cal) | gi 52 ▼ low

PORK, SOY & SNOWPEA SAN CHOY BOW

2 teaspoons vegetable oil
500 g (1 lb) lean pork mince
1 clove garlic, crushed
4 spring onions (scallions), sliced
200 g (6½ oz) can water
  chestnuts, drained
  weight 135 g (4½ oz)
300 g (10 oz) can soybeans,
  drained weight 220 g (7 oz)
200 g (6½ oz) snowpeas, sliced
2 tablespoons oyster sauce
8 iceberg lettuce leaves

1 Heat the oil in a wok, add pork mince and stir fry over medium heat for 5 minutes, or until browned.
2 Add the garlic and spring onions and cook for 2 minutes more or until the onions soften.
3 Add the water chestnuts, soybeans, snowpeas and oyster sauce and simmer for 10 minutes.
4 Serve bowls of the pork mixture accompanied by the lettuce leaves and allow each person to roll up their own leaves with the pork. Serves 4

per serve | fat 14.5 g | protein 32.5 g | carbohydrate 10.5 g | fibre 5.5 g | cholesterol 75 mg | energy 1250 kj (300 cal) | gi 24 ▼ low

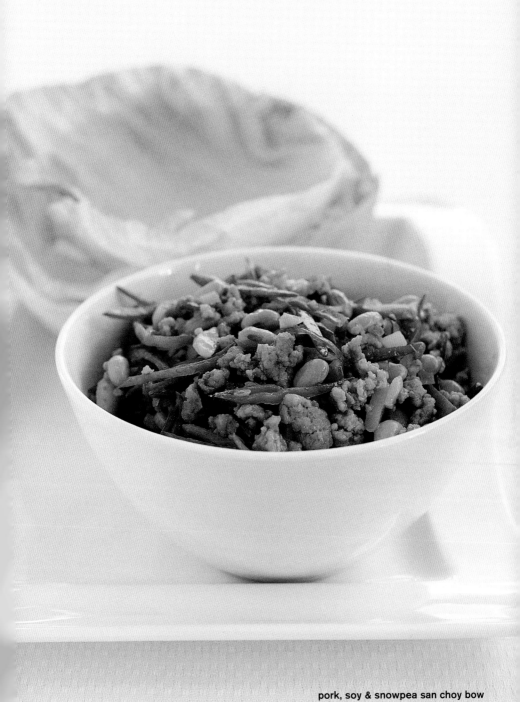

pork, soy & snowpea san choy bow

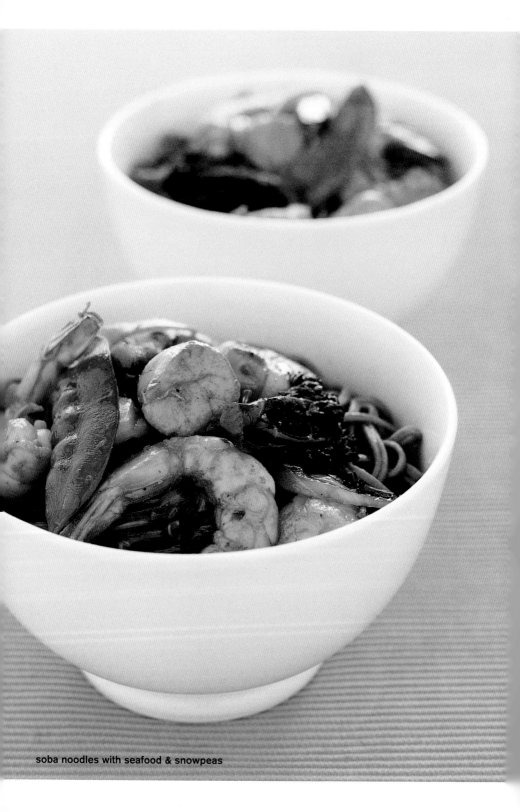

soba noodles with seafood & snowpeas

SOBA NOODLES WITH SEAFOOD & SNOWPEAS

1 Cook the soba noodles in a medium pan of cold water until they come to the boil, add another cup of water and stir until they return to the boil. Cook for 5 minutes or until tender. Drain well.
2 Heat the oil in a wok, add the garlic, ginger and onion and stir fry over medium heat for 3 minutes or until the onion is soft.
3 Add the seafood and stir fry over high heat for 3 minutes. Add the soy, honey, stock, lemon, snowpeas and broccolini or broccoli and stir fry for 3 minutes, or until the vegetables are just tender.
4 Serve nests of the noodles with the seafood mixture mounded on top. Serves 4

per serve | fat 4.5 g | protein 48.5 g | carbohydrate 64.5 g | fibre 10 g | cholesterol 267 mg | energy 1990 kj (475 cal) | gi 46 ▽ low

300 g (10 oz) dried soba noodles
2 teaspoons olive oil
2 cloves garlic, crushed
1 tablespoon grated fresh ginger
1 medium onion, thinly sliced
750 g (1½ lb) mixed, cleaned
   seafood (prawns, calamari,
   mussels, scallops)
1 tablespoon reduced-salt
   soy sauce
2 teaspoons honey
½ cup (125 ml/4 fl oz)
   reduced-salt fish stock
2 teaspoons grated lemon zest
200 g (6½ oz) snowpeas
1 bunch (200 g/6½ oz) broccolini
   or broccoli, chopped

TOFU, VEGETABLE & RICE NOODLE STIR FRY

1 Rinse the noodles under cold water to separate.
2 Cut the tofu into 2.5 cm (1 in) cubes. Heat the oils in a wok, add the ginger and tofu and stir fry over high heat for 3 minutes or until tofu is golden.
3 Add the carrot, corn and capsicum and stir fry for 3 minutes or until the vegetables are soft.
4 Add the bok choy, soy, stock and noodles and stir fry for 3 minutes or until heated through.
5 Remove from heat and toss through the bean sprouts. Serve hot. Serves 4

per serve | fat 13.5 g | protein 20 g | carbohydrate 60 g | fibre 6.5 g | cholesterol 0 mg | energy 1850 kj (440 cal) | gi 35 ▽ low

500 g (1 lb) fresh rice noodles
375 g (12 oz) firm tofu
1 teaspoon sesame oil
1 tablespoon vegetable oil
1 tablespoon grated fresh ginger
1 carrot, peeled and sliced
100 g (3⅓ oz) baby corn, halved
1 red capsicum (bell pepper),
   seeded and sliced
1 bunch (250 g/8 oz) baby bok
   choy, leaves separated
2 tablespoons reduced-salt
   soy sauce
½ cup (125 ml/4 fl oz)
   reduced-salt vegetable stock
1 cup (110 g/3½ oz) bean sprouts

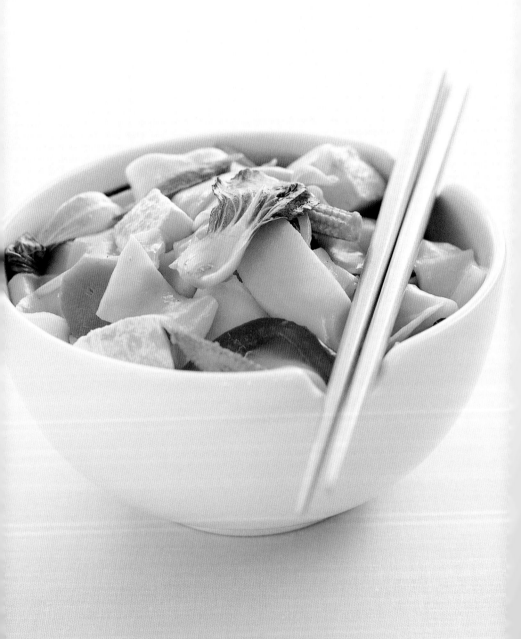

tofu, vegetable & rice noodle stir fry

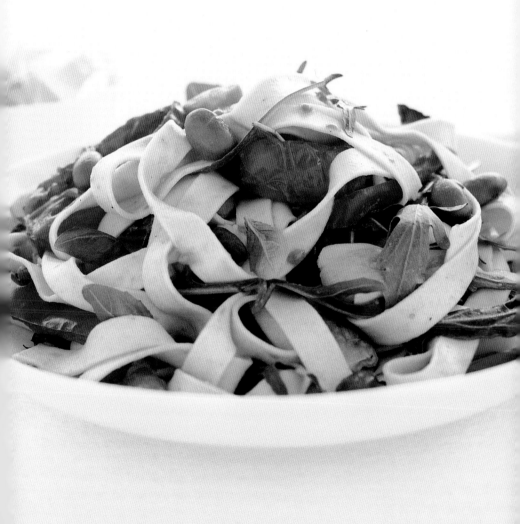

fettuccine with roast tomato & capsicum

FETTUCCINE WITH ROAST TOMATO & CAPSICUM

200 g (6½ oz) cherry tomatoes
6 (375 g/12 oz) Roma tomatoes
1 head garlic, separated into
   cloves but not peeled
1 red capsicum (bell pepper),
   seeded and cut into thin strips
olive oil spray
400 g (13 oz) fettuccine
½ cup (15 g/½ oz) fresh basil
400 g (13 oz) can borlotti beans,
   drained weight 300g (10 oz)
100 g (3⅓ oz) baby rocket
   (arugula)
½ cup (45 g/1½ oz) grated
   parmesan cheese, to serve

1 Preheat oven to 200°C (400°F/Gas 6).
2 Halve the cherry and Roma tomatoes and put with garlic and capsicum into a large baking dish. Spray lightly with olive oil spray and season with pepper.
3 Bake for 40 minutes or until the Roma tomatoes are soft. Peel the garlic and discard the skins.
4 Cook the pasta in a large pan of rapidly boiling water until al dente (cooked, but still with a bite to it). Drain well and return to the pan.
5 Add the roasted vegetables. Stir in the basil leaves, beans, rocket and parmesan and toss gently to combine. Serves 4

per serve | fat 4.5 g | protein 16.5 g | carbohydrate 62.5 g | fibre 7 g | cholesterol 6.5 mg | energy 1465 kj (350 cal) | gi 40 ▼ low

CHARGRILLED LAMB WITH WARM TABOULI

1½ cups (375 ml/12 fl oz)
   reduced-salt chicken stock
1 cup (180 g/6 oz) bulgur wheat
250 g (8 oz) cherry tomatoes, halved
1 cup (30 g/1 oz) chopped
   fresh flat-leaf parsley
½ cup (15 g/½ oz) chopped
   fresh mint
4 spring onions (scallions), sliced
1 tablespoon extra virgin olive oil
2 tablespoons lemon juice
500 g (1 lb) lean lamb loin
½ teaspoon ground allspice
8 vine leaves (200 g/6½ oz)
   preserved in brine
olive oil spray
200 g (6½ oz) low-fat hummus
250 g (8 oz) wholemeal pita bread

1 Put the stock into a pan and bring to the boil. Add bulgur wheat, reduce heat, cover and simmer for 15 minutes or until liquid is absorbed. Remove from the heat and set aside uncovered for 10 minutes.
2 Stir through the tomatoes, parsley, chopped mint, spring onions, olive oil and lemon and keep warm.
3 Rub the lamb with the allspice and wrap in the vine leaves. Cook on a lightly olive oil-sprayed, preheated chargrill for 3-5 minutes on each side, or until cooked to your liking.
4 Rest the lamb in a warm place for 5-10 minutes before slicing. Serve with warm tabouli, hummus and pita bread. Serves 6

per serve | fat 14 g | protein 28.5 g | carbohydrate 42 g | fibre 11.5 g | cholesterol 56.5 mg | energy 1725 kj (410 cal) | gi 49 ▼ low

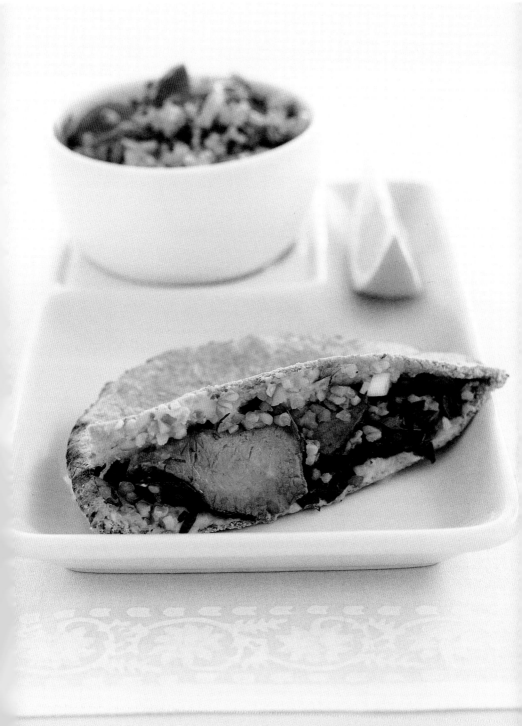

chargrilled lamb with warm tabouli

CHICKEN TAGINE WITH SPICED CHICKPEAS

2 teaspoons olive oil

8 (1.2 kg/2 lb 6½ oz) skinless
medium chicken drumsticks
(700 g/1 lb 6½ oz edible weight)

1 medium onion, sliced

¼ teaspoon saffron threads

330 g (11 oz) peeled orange
sweet potato, cut into chunks

2 medium zucchini (courgette),
cut into thick slices

1 tablespoon finely
shredded orange zest

100 g (3⅓ oz) dried apricots

100 g (3⅓ oz) dried prunes

400 g (13 oz) can chopped
tomatoes

2 cups (500 ml/16 fl oz)
reduced-salt chicken stock

1 cinnamon stick

195 g (6½ oz) pearl barley

400 g (13 oz) can chickpeas,
drained weight 300 g (10 oz)

2 tablespoons roughly chopped,
fresh flat-leaf parsley

1 Heat the oil in a large heatproof casserole dish or Dutch oven, add the chicken in batches and cook over medium heat for 3-5 minutes or until browned.

2 Return all the chicken to the pan, add the onion and saffron and cook for 5 minutes or until the onion is soft and translucent.

3 Add the sweet potato, zucchini, orange zest, dried fruit, tomatoes, stock and cinnamon stick.
Bring to the boil, reduce heat, cover and simmer gently for 40 minutes.

4 Remove the lid and cook for 10 minutes or until the chicken comes away from the bone.

5 While the chicken is cooking, put the barley into a pan, cover with 4 cups (1 litre/32 fl oz) water and bring to the boil. Simmer, uncovered, for 25 minutes.

6 Add the chickpeas to the barley and cook for 5 minutes more, or until both are tender. Drain well, then stir in the parsley. Serve mounds of the barley mixture topped with the tagine. Serves 8

per serve | fat 8.5 g | protein 24 g | carbohydrate 41.5 g | fibre 8 g | cholesterol 88.5 mg | energy 1405kj (335 cal) | gi 33 ▼ low

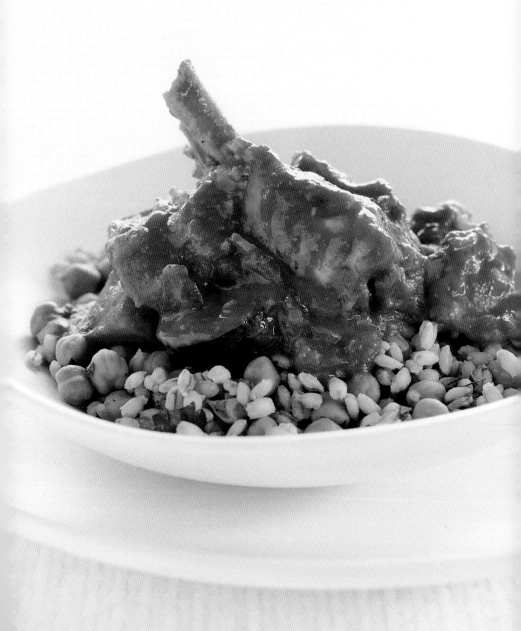

chicken tagine with spiced chickpeas

LEMON HERB TUNA WITH RICE & LENTILS

1 cup (190 g/6¼ oz) brown
   lentils, soaked in cold
   water overnight
1 tablespoon olive oil
4 medium onions, thinly sliced
¼ cup (60 ml/2 fl oz)
   reduced-salt chicken stock
1 cup (205 g/6½ oz) basmati rice
4 (630 g/1¼ lb) trimmed
   tuna steaks
olive oil spray
½ cup (15 g/½ oz) chopped
   fresh flat-leaf parsley
½ cup (15g/½ oz) chopped
   fresh coriander (cilantro)
3 cloves garlic, crushed
1 teaspoon ground cumin
1 teaspoon paprika
juice and zest of 1 lemon
2 tablespoons fat-free dressing

1 Drain and rinse the lentils and discard any small stones. Put in a medium pan and just cover with water. Bring to the boil, reduce heat and simmer for 10 minutes, then drain well.

2 Heat the oil in a large, deep fry pan, add the onion and cook over medium heat for 5 minutes or until soft. Add the stock and cook for 10 minutes more, or until the stock evaporates and the onions brown.

3 Add the rice, lentils and 3 cups (750 ml/24 fl oz) water, bring to the boil and simmer for 5 minutes or until tunnels appear on the surface. Cover with foil, reduce the heat to low and cook for 10-15 minutes more or until the rice is soft.

4 Cook the tuna on a lightly olive oil-sprayed, preheated chargrill pan for 2-3 minutes on each side, or according to your preference.

5 Put the parsley, coriander, garlic, spices, lemon juice, zest and dressing into a bowl and whisk to combine. Serve the tuna drizzled with herb sauce and rice to the side. Serves 4

per serve | fat 14.5 g | protein 57 g | carbohydrate 65 g | fibre 10 g | cholesterol 57 mg | energy 2600 kj (620 cal) | gi 45 ▼ low

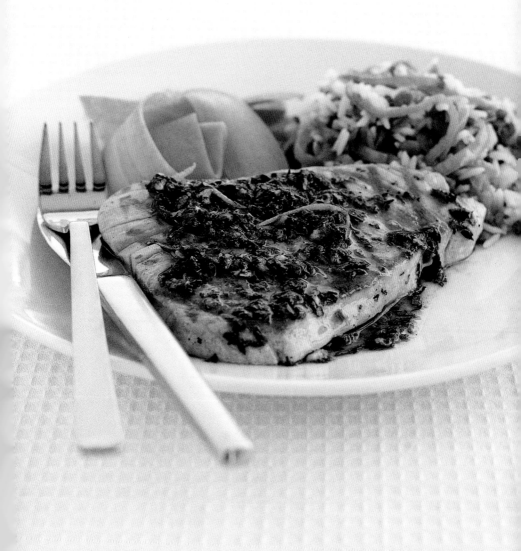

lemon herb tuna with rice & lentils

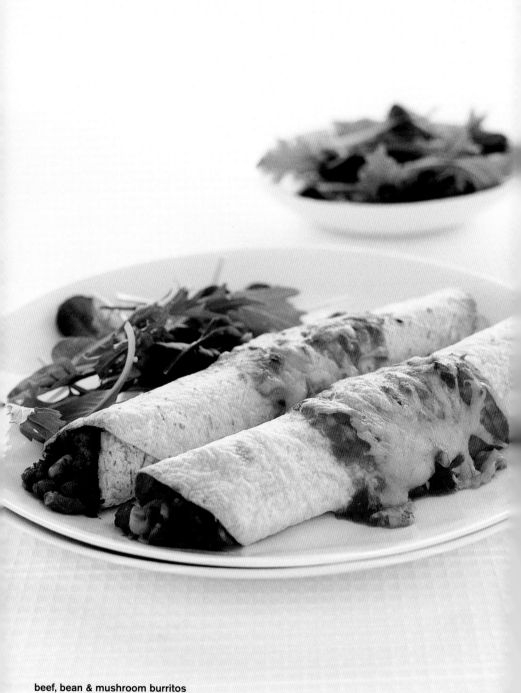

beef, bean & mushroom burritos

BEEF, BEAN & MUSHROOM BURRITOS

1 Heat the oil in a large fry pan, add the onion and cook over medium heat for 3 minutes or until the onion is soft.

2 Add the mince and cook for 5 minutes until browned. Add the capsicum and mushrooms and cook for about 5 minutes or until soft.

3 Add the beans, tomatoes and corn, bring to the boil and simmer for 15 minutes or until sauce has thickened slightly. Stir in the coriander.

4 Spread some of the meat mixture down the center of a tortilla and roll up to enclose filling.

5 Arrange the rolled tortillas in a large ovenproof dish. Spoon the salsa evenly over the top and sprinkle with grated cheese.

6 Bake for 20 minutes or until the cheese is golden. Serve with a mixed green salad. Serves 6

per serve | fat 10.5 g | protein 25.5 g | carbohydrate 45.5 g | fibre 9.5 g | cholesterol 32.5 mg | energy 1590 kj (380 cal) | gi 36 ▼ low

2 teaspoons olive oil

1 medium onion, chopped

350 g (12 oz) lean beef mince

1 red capsicum (bell pepper), seeded and chopped

1 green capsicum (bell pepper), seeded and chopped

300 g (10 oz) mushrooms, sliced

400 g (13 oz) can ready-made chilli beans

400 g (13 oz) can chopped tomatoes

1 cup (200 g/6½ oz) fresh or frozen corn kernels

2 tablespoons chopped fresh coriander (cilantro)

8 flour tortillas, 20 cm (8 in) in diameter

1½ cups (375 g/12 oz) mild bottled tomato salsa

¼ cup (30 g/1 oz) grated reduced-fat cheddar cheese

LAMB SHANKS, MUSHY PEAS & GRAVY

1 tablespoon olive oil

4 (540 g/1 lb 1⅓ oz trimmed
   weight) Frenched lamb shanks

8 pickling onions, peeled
   and left whole

2 cloves garlic, crushed

2 cups (500 ml/16 fl oz)
   reduced-salt beef stock

½ cup (125 ml/4 fl oz) red wine

1 bay leaf

4 black peppercorns

200 g (6½ oz) peeled baby carrots

3⅔ cups (500 g/1 lb) frozen peas

20 g (⅔ oz) reduced-fat
   polyunsaturated margarine

1 Heat the oil in a large heatproof casserole dish or Dutch oven. Add the lamb shanks in batches and cook over medium heat until browned all over. Return all the lamb to the pan.

2 Add the onions and cook for 3-5 minutes or until browned, then add the garlic and stir. Add the stock, red wine, bay leaf and peppercorns. Cover and simmer gently for 45 minutes.

3 Add whole carrots and cook for 15 minutes more, or until carrots are tender and the lamb comes away from the bone. Remove the lamb, carrots and onions, cover and keep warm.

4 Increase the heat, boil liquid for 10 minutes or until reduced and thickened slightly.

5 Put the peas into a pan, cover with water, bring to the boil and simmer for 10 minutes or until tender. Drain well and add the margarine, then roughly mash together with the peas.

6 Serve the lamb shanks and vegetables with a mound of mashed peas and drizzle the sauce over the top. Serves 4

per serve | **fat 9.5 g** | **protein 40.5 g** | **carbohydrate 18.5 g** | **fibre 9.5 g** | **cholesterol 84 mg** | **energy 1440 kj (345 cal)** | **gi 38** ▽ **low**

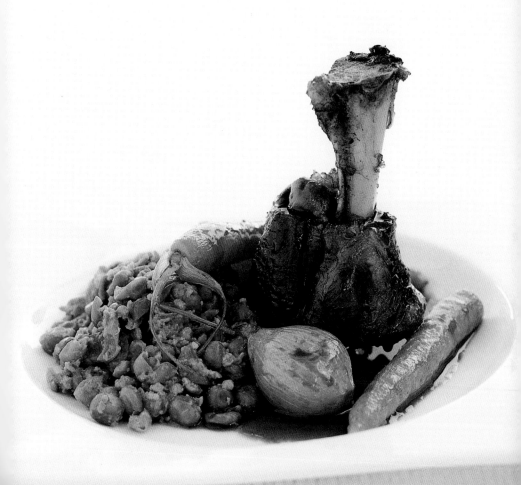

lamb shanks, mushy peas & gravy

SWEET THINGS

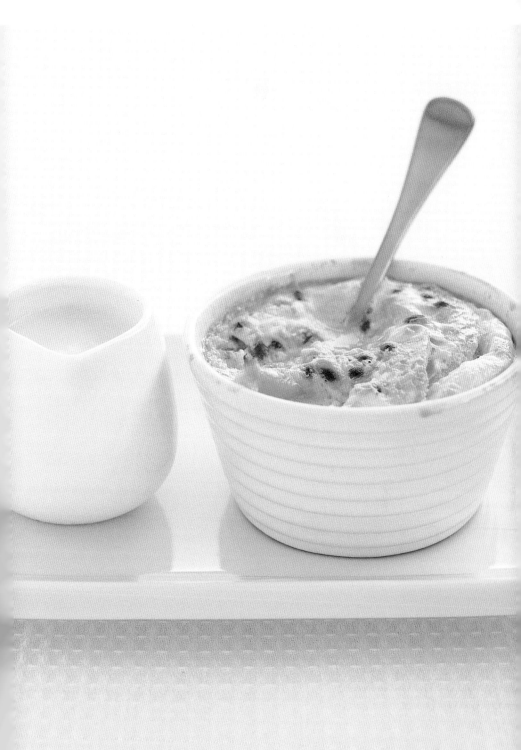

baked mango & passionfruit custards

BAKED MANGO & PASSIONFRUIT CUSTARDS

150 g (5 oz) mango flesh,
thinly sliced
1 cup (250 ml/8 fl oz)
reduced-fat milk
3 eggs, lightly beaten
¼ cup (60 g/2 oz) caster sugar
or low-calorie sweetener
suitable for cooking
½ cup (125 ml/4 fl oz)
passionfruit pulp

1 Preheat oven to 180°C (350°F/Gas 4).
2 Arrange the mango slices in the bases of
4 x ½ cup (125 ml/4 fl oz) capacity ramekins.
3 Whisk together the milk, eggs, sugar or sweetener
and passionfruit and pour over the mango.
4 Bake the custards for 20 minutes or until they
are just set. Serve warm. Serves 4

per serve (sugar) | fat 5 g | protein 8.5 g
| carbohydrate 23 g | fibre 5 g | cholesterol 145 mg
| energy 710 kj (170 cal) | gi 56 ◆ med
per serve (sweetener) | fat 5 g | protein 8.5 g
| carbohydrate 11.5 g | fibre 5 g | cholesterol 145 mg
| energy 525 kj (125 cal) | gi 37 ▼ low

SEMOLINA CAKE WITH VANILLA PEARS

1 cup (140 g/4½ oz)
self-raising flour
1½ cups (240 g/7⅔ oz) semolina
⅓ cup (80 g/2 ⅔ oz) caster
sugar or low-calorie sweetener
suitable for cooking
2 teaspoons finely grated
lemon zest
3 eggs, lightly beaten
200 ml (6½ fl oz) no-fat,
no-added sugar vanilla yoghurt
60 g (2 oz) reduced-fat
polyunsaturated margarine
4 medium pears, unpeeled,
uncored and sliced lengthwise
1½ cups (375 ml/12 fl oz)
unsweetened apple juice
1 vanilla bean, halved lengthwise
400 ml (13 fl oz) no-fat, no-added
sugar vanilla yoghurt, to serve

1 Preheat oven to 180°C (350°F/Gas 4). Lightly
grease and line a 20 cm (8 in) spring form tin.
2 Sift the flour and semolina into a bowl and stir in
sugar or sweetener and zest. Whisk together the
eggs, yoghurt and melted margarine and mix into
the dry ingredients until smooth. Pour into the tin.
3 Bake for 40-50 minutes or until a skewer comes
out clean when inserted into the center. Cool in
the tin for 5 minutes then turn out on a wire rack.
4 Put the pears, apple juice and vanilla bean into
a pan and bring to the boil. Reduce heat, cover and
simmer for 10 minutes or until the pears are just soft.
5 Serve wedges of the cake with poached pears,
poaching liquid and yoghurt. Serves 10

per serve (sugar) | fat 5 g | protein 9.5 g
| carbohydrate 49 g | fibre 3 g | cholesterol 61 mg
| energy 1175 kj (280 cal) | gi 51 ▼ low
per serve (sweetener) | fat 5 g | protein 9.5 g
| carbohydrate 42 g | fibre 3 g | cholesterol 61 mg
| energy 1060 kj (255 cal) | gi 49 ▼ low

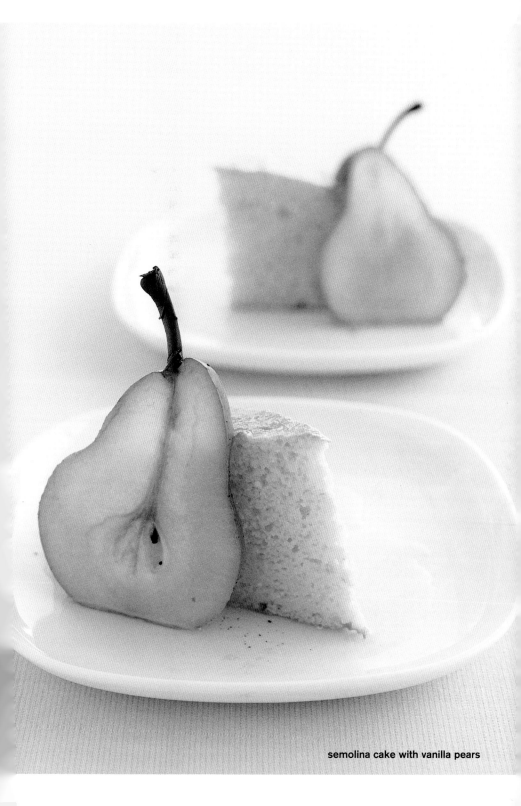

semolina cake with vanilla pears

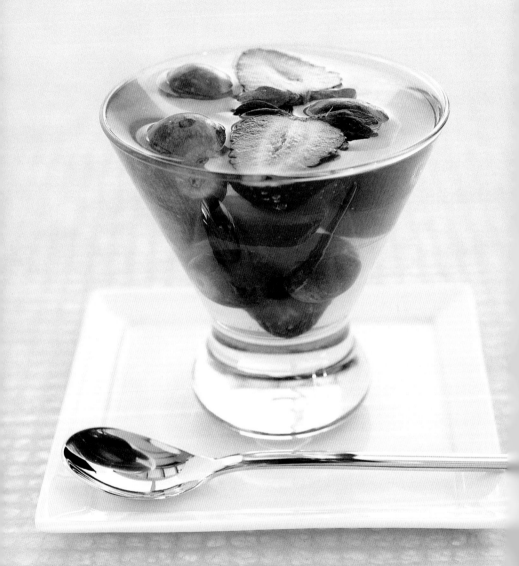

apple & grape jellies

APPLE & GRAPE JELLIES

1 Put the gelatin and apple juice into a pan and stir over low heat for about 2 minutes or until the gelatin dissolves. Remove from the heat and cool slightly.
2 Divide ⅓ cup (90 g/3 oz) of the fruit among 4 x 1 cup (250 ml/8 fl oz) capacity glasses.
3 Pour in enough of the apple liquid to cover the fruit, cover and chill the glasses for 20 minutes or until the jelly is just set.
4 Divide the remaining berries and grapes among the glasses, pour over the remaining liquid and chill for 4 hours or until set. Serves 4

per serve | **fat 0 g** | **protein 4 g** | **carbohydrate 32.5 g** | **fibre 1 g** | **cholesterol 0 mg** | **energy 595 kj (140 cal)** | **gi 41** ▼ **low**

4 teaspoons gelatin
3 cups (750 ml/24 fl oz)
  unsweetened apple juice
100 g (3⅓ oz) strawberries,
  cut into halves
300 g (10 oz) seedless green
  or black grapes

PEACH & GRAPEFRUIT GRANITA WITH CITRUS

1 Put the sugar or sweetener, grapefruit juice, sliced peaches and juice into a pan. Stir over low heat until the sugar dissolves.
2 Pour into a shallow non-reactive metal container. Freeze until the mixture starts to harden around the edges, then break up the crystals with a fork.
3 Return to the freezer for 1 hour, break up with a fork, repeat the whole process and freeze again.
4 Put the segmented oranges, grapefruit, tangerines and orange flower water into a non-metallic bowl and mix to combine.
5 Serve the granita in chilled glasses with citrus salad to the side. Serves 6

per serve (sugar) | **fat 0.5 g** | **protein 2.5 g** | **carbohydrate 30 g** | **fibre 3 g** | **cholesterol 0 mg** | **energy 575 kj (140 cal)** | **gi 44** ▼ **low**
per serve (sweetener) | **fat 0.5 g** | **protein 2.5 g** | **carbohydrate 25 g** | **fibre 3 g** | **cholesterol 0 mg** | **energy 495 kj (120 cal)** | **gi 38** ▼ **low**

2 tablespoons caster sugar
  or low-calorie sweetener
  suitable for cooking
3 cups (750 ml/24 fl oz) pink
  grapefruit juice, unsweetened
400 g (13 oz) can peaches in juice
2 medium navel oranges,
  cut into segments
3 pink grapefruit, segmented
2 tangerines, segmented
1 teaspoon orange flower water

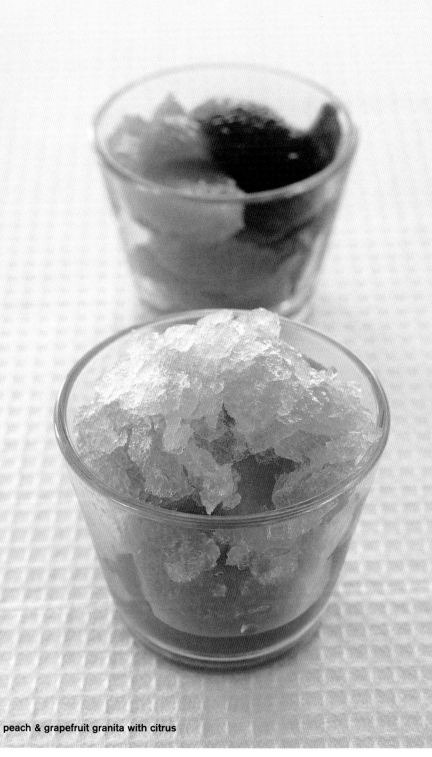

peach & grapefruit granita with citrus

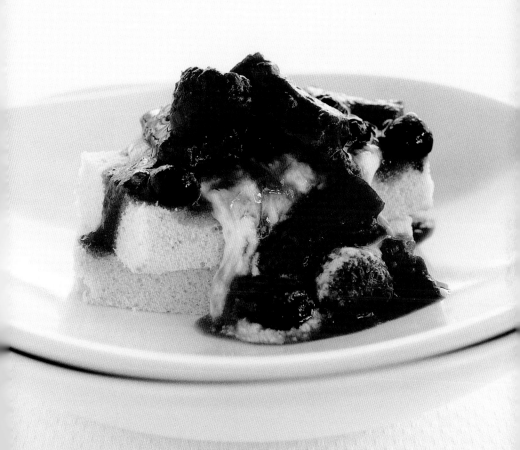

rhubarb & mixed berry ricotta sponge

RHUBARB & MIXED BERRY RICOTTA SPONGE

1 bunch (330 g/11 oz) rhubarb,
leaves discarded

¼ cup (60 ml/2 fl oz)
unsweetened apple juice

2 tablespoons caster sugar
or low-calorie sweetener
suitable for cooking

200 g (6½ oz) fresh or
frozen mixed berries

200 g (6½ oz) prepared
plain sponge cake

100 g (3⅓ oz) low-fat
ricotta cheese

200 ml (6½ fl oz) no-fat, no-added
sugar vanilla yoghurt

1 Preheat oven to 180°C (350°F/Gas 4).

2 Wash the rhubarb and cut into 5 cm (2 in) pieces. Put in a pan with apple juice and sugar or sweetener and stir over low heat until sugar dissolves.

3 Cover and cook for 5 minutes, then add the berries, cover and cook for a further 5 minutes or until the rhubarb is soft.

4 Cut the sponge cake into 8 even slices. Put the ricotta and yoghurt into a bowl and mix to combine.

5 Arrange 2 sponge slices on each plate and top with the ricotta mixture and stewed fruit. Serves 4

per serve (sugar) ⎮ **fat 3 g** ⎮ **protein 8.5 g** ⎮ **carbohydrate 19 g** ⎮ **fibre 4 g** ⎮ **cholesterol 41.5 mg** ⎮ **energy 590 kj (140 cal)** ⎮ **gi 49** ▼ **low**

per serve (sweetener) ⎮ **fat 3 g** ⎮ **protein 8.5 g** ⎮ **carbohydrate 11.5 g** ⎮ **fibre 4 g** ⎮ **cholesterol 41.5 mg** ⎮ **energy 475 kj (115 cal)** ⎮ **gi 32** ▼ **low**

LOW-FAT ICE CREAM CASSATA SLICE

300 g (10 oz) low-fat chocolate
ice cream, softened

⅓ cup (50 g/1⅔ oz) pine nuts,
roughly chopped

250 g (8 oz) low-fat vanilla ice
cream, softened

100 g (3⅓ oz) dried apricots,
roughly chopped

100 g (3⅓ oz) dried figs, chopped

100 g (3⅓ oz) dried peaches,
roughly chopped

50 g (1⅔ oz) red and green
glacé cherries, chopped

1 Line a 20 cm x 10 cm (8 in x 4 in) bar tin with enough plastic wrap to hang down the sides of the tin.

2 Put the chocolate ice cream and pine nuts into a bowl and mix to combine. Spoon the mixture into the base and up the sides of the tin, leaving the center hollow. Freeze until firm.

3 Mix the vanilla ice cream with the dried fruit and spoon into the bar tin over the chocolate ice cream. Smooth the surface and cover with overhanging plastic wrap. Freeze overnight or until firm.

5 Remove from the tin, discard the plastic and slice with a knife heated under hot water. Serves 6

per serve ⎮ **fat 6.5 g** ⎮ **protein 5.5 g** ⎮ **carbohydrate 35 g** ⎮ **fibre 4.5 g** ⎮ **cholesterol 7 mg** ⎮ **energy 910 kj (220 cal)** ⎮ **gi 44** ▼ **low**

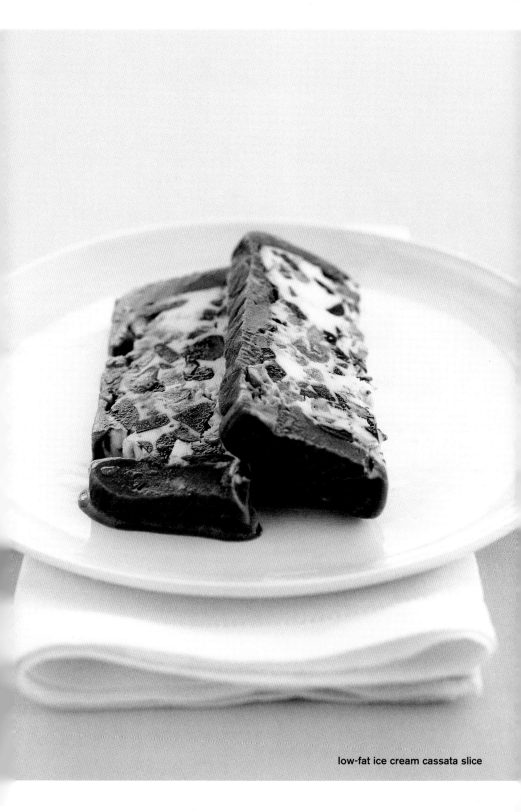

low-fat ice cream cassata slice

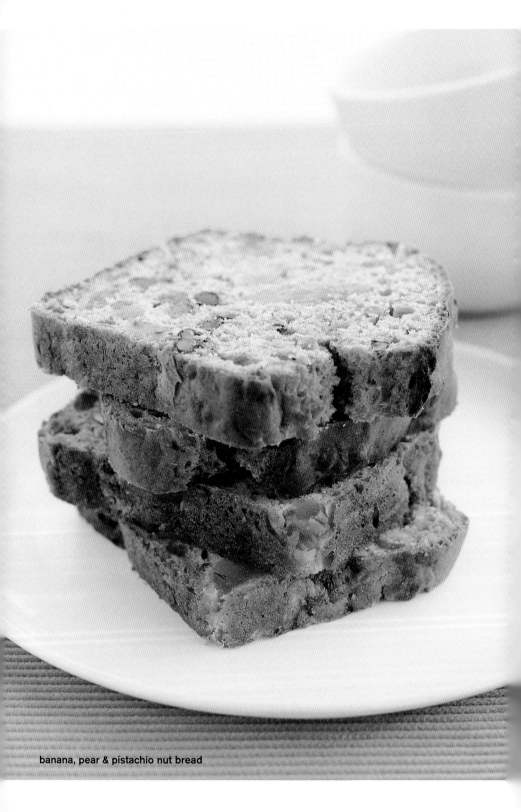

banana, pear & pistachio nut bread

BANANA, PEAR & PISTACHIO NUT BREAD

1 Preheat oven to 180°C (350°F/Gas 4). Grease and line a 20 cm x 10 cm (8 in x 4 in) loaf tin.
2 Put the pears into a bowl and just cover with boiling water for 10 minutes or until soft. Drain well.
3 Sift the flours, baking powder and cinnamon into a bowl. Stir in the sugar or sweetener and nuts.
4 Whisk together the eggs, buttermilk and oil and stir through the dry ingredients, banana and pears.
5 Spoon the mixture into the prepared tin and bake for 55-60 minutes or until a skewer comes out clean when inserted into the center.
6 Cool in the tin for 5 minutes, then turn out on a wire rack to cool before slicing. Serves 10

per serve (sugar) | fat 8 g | protein 7.5 g
| carbohydrate 47.5 g | fibre 4.5 g | cholesterol 40 mg
| energy 1215 kj (290 cal) | gi 55 ▼ low

per serve (sweetener) | fat 8 g | protein 7.5 g
| carbohydrate 44.5 g | fibre 4.5 g | cholesterol 40 mg
| energy 1165 kj (280 cal) | gi 54 ▼ low

200 g (6½ oz) dried pears,
  roughly chopped
2¼ cups (280 g/8 oz)
  self-raising flour
70 g (2⅓ oz) plain flour
1 teaspoon baking powder
1 teaspoon ground cinnamon
3 tablespoons brown sugar
  or low-calorie sweetener
  suitable for cooking
⅓ cup (50 g/1⅔ oz) pistachio
  nuts, chopped
2 eggs, lightly beaten
1 cup (250 ml/8 fl oz) buttermilk
2 tablespoons vegetable oil
1 cup (240 g/7⅔ oz) mashed
  ripe banana

POACHED SAFFRON FRUIT POTS WITH FILO

1 Preheat oven to 200°C (400°F/Gas 6).
2 Put the dried fruit, saffron, cinnamon, orange juice, zest and apple juice into a pan. Bring to the boil, reduce heat, cover and simmer for 10 minutes or until the fruit is soft. Spoon the mixture into 6 x 1 cup (250 ml/8 fl oz) capacity ramekins.
3 Brush each of the filo sheets with melted margarine, cut into 6 equal squares and scrunch into 24 balls. Arrange on top of the fruit.
4 Bake for 10 minutes or until the pastry is crisp and golden. Serve immediately. Serves 6

per serve | fat 2 g | protein 4 g | carbohydrate 62 g
| fibre 10.5 g | cholesterol 0 mg | energy 1145 kj
(275 cal) | gi 38 ▼ low

200 g (6½ oz) dried apricots
200 g (6½ oz) dried pears
100 g (3⅓ oz) dried figs
100 g (3⅓ oz) dried prunes
pinch saffron threads
1 cinnamon stick
juice and zest of 1 orange
1 cup (250 ml/8 fl oz)
  unsweetened apple juice
4 sheets filo (phyllo) pastry
10 g (⅓ oz) reduced-fat
  polyunsaturated margarine

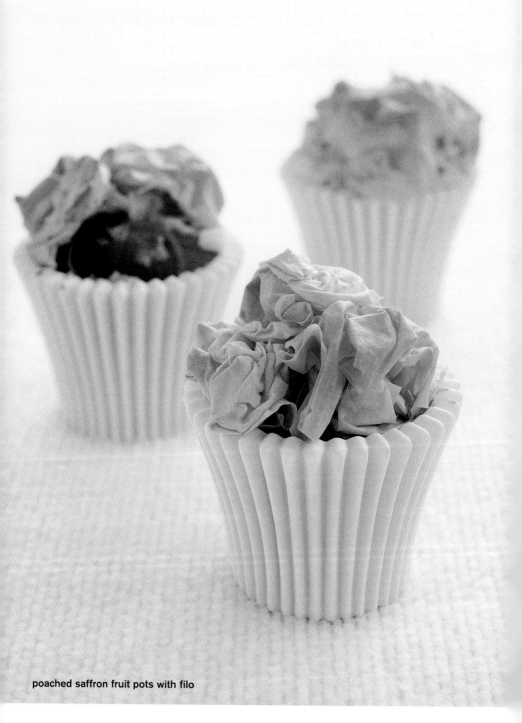

poached saffron fruit pots with filo

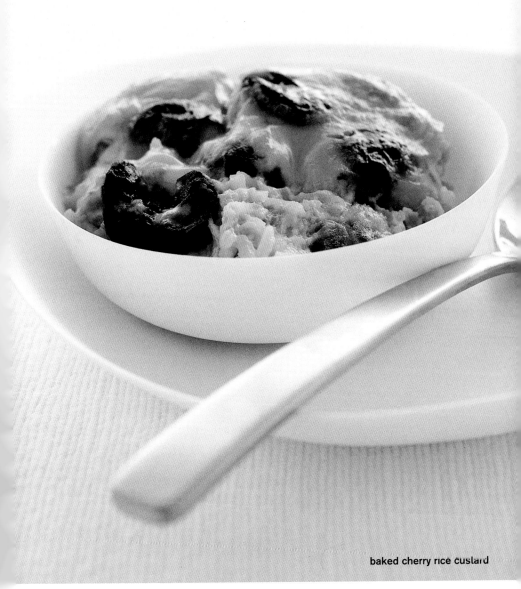

baked cherry rice custard

BAKED CHERRY RICE CUSTARD

3 tablespoons basmati rice

2 cups (500 ml/16 fl oz) water

3 eggs, lightly beaten

2 tablespoons caster sugar

1 teaspoon vanilla essence

2½ cups (625 ml/20 fl oz) skim
or no-fat milk

400 g (13 oz) can pitted cherries,
drained weight 280 g (9 oz)

1 Preheat oven to 180°C (350°F/Gas 4).

2 Put the rice and water into a pan, boil uncovered for 10 minutes then drain well. Whisk together the eggs, sugar, vanilla and milk. Add rice and mix.

3 Pour into a 4 cup (1 litre/32 fl oz) capacity ovenproof dish and scatter cherries over the top.

4 Put the dish into a deep baking tray. Pour hot water into the tray until it is halfway up the dish sides. Bake for 50 minutes or until set. Serves 6

per serve | fat 2.5 g | protein 8 g | carbohydrate 25.5 g | fibre 1g | cholesterol 97 mg | energy 660 kj (160 cal) | gi 45 ▼ low

QUICK-MIX FRUIT CAKE

350 g (12 oz) mixed dried fruit

2 cups (340 g/11¼ oz) sultanas

1 cup (135 g/4½ oz) dried
apricots, chopped

⅔ cup (80 g/2⅔ oz) blanched
almonds, chopped

125 g (4 oz) reduced-fat
polyunsaturated margarine

½ cup (115 g/3⅔ oz) brown
sugar or low-calorie sweetener
suitable for cooking

1½ cups (375 ml/12 fl oz)
unsweetened apple juice

¾ cup (105 g/3½ oz) stone
ground plain flour

105 g (3½ oz) self-raising flour

2 teaspoons mixed spice

2 eggs, lightly beaten

2 cups (500 ml/16 fl oz)
low-fat custard

1 Preheat oven to 160°C (315°F/Gas 2½). Grease and line a 20 cm (8 in) round cake tin with two layers of baking paper.

2 Put the fruit, almonds, margarine, sugar or sweetener and apple juice into a pan and simmer for 2 minutes. Transfer to a bowl and cool.

3 Sift flours and spice into a bowl, add the eggs and fruit and mix to combine. Spoon mixture into the tin and smooth the top down with wet fingers.

4 Wrap several layers of newspaper around the outside of the tin and secure it with kitchen string.

5 Bake the cake for 1½-2 hours or until a skewer comes out clean when inserted into the center. Cool briefly in the tin, then turn out on a wire rack. Serve warm with custard or cold. Makes 16 slices

per serve (sugar) | fat 8 g | protein 6 g | carbohydrate 58 g | fibre 4 g | cholesterol 25.5 mg | energy 1340 kj (320 cal) | gi 49 ▼ low

per serve (sweetener) | fat 8 g | protein 6 g | carbohydrate 51.5 g | fibre 4 g | cholesterol 25.5 mg | energy 1240 kj (295 cal) | gi 46 ▼ low

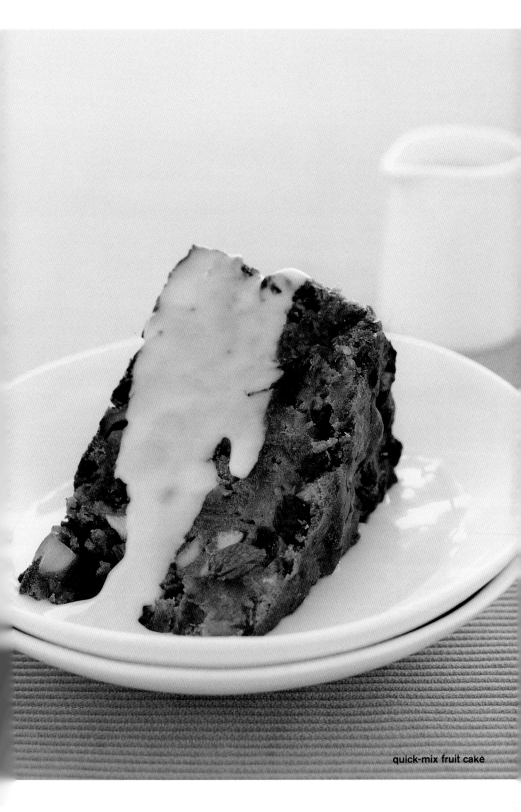

quick-mix fruit cake

antioxidant - a substance that prevents body tissues from being damaged by oxidation caused by free radicals, which are thought to be associated with many disease processes and are formed in the body naturally or from exposure to pollution, cigarette smoking, chemicals and the sun.

carbohydrates - a group of nutrients that includes starches, sugars and fibres. All carbohydrates, except for fibres, are made up of sugar units. They are broken down into sugars during digestion. Different carbohydrates are made up of chains of sugars bound together in different ways. They are both digested and their sugar absorbed into the blood at different rates (see glycaemic index on pages 6-7).

glucose - a type of sugar that makes up the starches and some sugars found in foods. Starches are broken down into glucose during digestion, which is then absorbed into the bloodstream and becomes blood glucose (blood sugar), the main fuel for the brain and muscles.

hypoglycaemia - the term for a lower than normal blood glucose level, often called a 'hypo'. It can be due to taking too much insulin or diabetes medication; not eating enough carbohydrate or missing a meal; drinking alcohol without food; or stress or extra exercise. Symptoms include feeling cold and weak, sweating, shakiness, irritability, confusion, and dizziness, and if blood sugar continues to fall it can lead to unconsciousness and coma.

insulin - a hormone secreted by the pancreas in response to rising blood sugar, which enables body cells to take up glucose from the blood, causing the blood glucose level to drop back down to normal. It also stimulates cells to take up fats and proteins from the blood.

omega-3 essential fats - polyunsaturated fats that have to be obtained from the diet because they cannot be made in the body. They are found in walnuts, linseed, canola oil, and oily fish like tuna, salmon, trout and mackerel. Increasing the intake of omega-3 fats while reducing saturated fat intake can help improve insulin action, reduce blood pressure and promote good circulation.

sweeteners and sugar substitutes - these can be either: 1. Nutritive sweeteners, which contain calories and increase blood sugar (eg, sugar, corn syrup, fructose, glucose, honey, maltose, fruit juice concentrate); 2. Sugar alcohols, which contain fewer calories and have a lower blood sugar response (eg, sorbitol, mannitol, isomalt); or 3. Non-nutritive or low-calorie sweeteners which are far sweeter than sugar and used in tiny amounts, so they provide almost no calories and won't increase blood sugar (eg, aspartame, acesulfame-K, Splenda®). Many 'lite' or reduced-sugar versions of sweet foods, such as soft drinks and jam, contain sugar alcohols and/or low-calorie sweeteners and can usually be consumed in moderation by people with diabetes.

Publisher Jody Vassallo
General manager Claire Connolly
Production manager Liz Fitzgerald
Recipes & styling Jody Vassallo
Photographer Ben Dearnley
Home economist Angela Treggoning
Recipe tester Camilla Jessop
Props stylist Melissa Singer
Designer Nicole Vonwiller
Editor Lynelle Scott-Aitken
Consulting nutritionist Dr Susanna Holt

STYLING CREDITS:
Lincraft (03) 9525 8770
Made in Japan (02) 9410 3799
Mud Australia (02) 9518 0220
Orson & Blake (02) 9326 1155
Royal Doulton (02) 9499 1904
Tomkin (02) 9319 2993
Villeroy & Boch (02) 9975 3099
Wheel & Barrow (02) 9413 9530
© **Recipes** Jody Vassallo 2002
© **Photography** Ben Dearnley
© **Series design** Fortiori Publishing

PUBLISHED BY FORTIORI PUBLISHING:
PO Box 3126 Nunawading
Victoria 3131 Australia
Phone: 61 3 9872 3855
Fax: 61 3 9872 5454
salesenquiries@fortiori.com.au
www.fortiori.com.au
order direct on (03) 9872 3855

First printed 2003. Reprinted 2004, 2006.
Printed by Toppan Printing Co (Aust) Pty Ltd.

ISBN 0 9581609 0 2

DISCLAIMER: The nutritional information listed under each recipe does not include the nutrient content of garnishes or any accompaniments not listed in specific quantities in the ingredient list. The nutritional information for each recipe is an estimate only, and may vary depending on the brand of ingredients used, and due to natural biological variations in the composition of natural foods such as meat, fish, fruit and vegetables. The nutritional information was calculated by a qualified dietitian using FoodWorks dietary analysis software (Version 3, Xyris Software Pty Ltd, Highgate Hill, Queensland, Australia) based on the Australian food composition tables and food manufacturers' data. Where not specified, ingredients are always analysed as average or medium, not small or large. All recipes were analysed using 59 g eggs.

IMPORTANT: Those who might be at risk from the effects of salmonella food poisoning (the elderly, pregnant women, young children and those suffering from immune deficiency diseases) should consult their general practitioner about consuming raw or undercooked eggs.